Survey Methods for Medical and Health Professions Education

Step	Finer Points

1) Needs Assessment	Confirm survey is appropriate method
	Find background information and prior surveys.
	Determine the best survey method:
	    Questionnaire
	    Interview
	    Focus group
	Narrow the topic.

2) Survey Construction	Create items for questionnaires or questions for interviews/focus groups.
3) Establishing Evidence	Collect validity and reliability evidence.
4) Survey Delivery	Determine the best survey medium (e.g., online). Adjust delivery to counter low response rates.
5) Data Analysis	Analyze individual items. Analyze scales. Evaluate for nonresponse bias.
6) Reporting Guidelines	Describe survey design and development efforts Report quantitative and qualitative findings cohesively per reporting guidelines.

Survey Methods for Medical and Health Professions Education

A Six-Step Approach

ANDREW W. PHILLIPS, MD, MEd

Adjunct Assistant Professor
Founder, EM Coach
Uniformed Services University

STEVEN J. DURNING, MD, PhD

Director, Center for Health Professions Education
Professor and Vice Chair, Department of Medicine
Uniformed Services University

ANTHONY R. ARTINO, Jr., PhD

Professor
School of Medicine and Health Sciences
The George Washington University

ELSEVIER

Elsevier
1600 John F. Kennedy Blvd.
Ste 1800
Philadelphia, PA 19103-2899

SURVEY METHODS FOR MEDICAL AND
HEALTH PROFESSIONS EDUCATION: A SIX-STEP APPROACH

ISBN: 978-0-323-69591-6

Library of Congress Control Number: 2021933306

Publisher: Elyse O'Grady
Senior Content Development Specialist: Angie Breckon
Publishing Services Manager: Shereen Jameel
Project Manager: Manikandan Chandrasekaran
Cover Design and Design Direction: Brian Salisbury

Printed in the United States of America

Last digit is the print number: 9 8 7 6 5 4 3 2

Working together
to grow libraries in
developing countries

www.elsevier.com • www.bookaid.org

To my father, Joe, my first editor, who has always been graciously relentless with his red pen. To my mother, Christina, for her endless support. To my wife, Cara, and my children, Luke and Sophia, for your sacrifices so I could edit this book. And to Drs. Christopher Straus, Barrett Fromme, Sandy Smith, Gus Garmel, Vineet Arora, and Shalini Reddy, my first mentors in the rewarding calling of medical education.

—*Andrew W. Phillips, MD, MEd*

To my wife, Kristen, and sons for their continuous love and support. To the many students, residents, colleagues, and patients who make the work of health professions education the privilege that it is.

—*Steven J. Durning, MD, PhD*

To my amazing, supportive family—Teri, Isabella, Tre, Jack, and Aiden—you are my love and my life; your encouragement and unconditional love nourish and sustain me. To my colleagues at the Uniformed Services University of the Health Sciences (USU)—virtually everything I know about health professions education I learned from the amazing leaders and scholars at USU. Thank you. And finally, to my new colleagues at the George Washington University School of Medicine and Health Sciences—I look forward to our future research and scholarship. The best is yet to come!

—*Anthony R. Artino, Jr., PhD*

Anthony R. Artino, Jr., PhD
Professor, George Washington University
   School of Medicine and Health Sciences
Washington, DC

Anna T. Cianciolo, PhD
Associate Professor, Department of Medical
   Education
Southern Illinois University School of
   Medicine
Springfield, Illinois

Jennifer A. Cleland, PhD
Professor of Medical Education Research
Vice-Dean of Education
Lee Kong Chian School of Medicine, Nayang
   Technological University Singapore

David A. Cook, MD, MHPE
Professor of Medicine and Medical
   Education
Mayo Clinic College of Medicine and
   Science
Director of Education Science
Office of Applied Scholarship and Education
   Science
Research Chair
Mayo Rochester Simulation Center
Rochester, Minnesota

Erik W. Driessen, PhD
Professor
Faculty of Health, Medicine, and Life sciences
School of Health Professions Education
Maastricht University
The Netherlands

Steven J. Durning, MD, PhD
Professor and Vice Chair of Medicine
Uniformed Services University
Director, Center for Health Professions
   Education
Bethesda, Maryland

Jeffrey LaRochelle, MD, MPH
Professor of Medicine
Assistant Dean of Medical Education
University of Central Florida College of
   Medicine
Orlando, Florida

Brian E. Mavis, PhD
Professor
Office of Medical Education Research and
   Development
Michigan State University College of Human
   Medicine
East Lansing, Michigan

Andrew W. Phillips, MD, MEd
Adjunct Assistant Professor
Uniformed Services University
Founder, EM Coach
Bethesda, Maryland

Amudha Poobalan, MBBS, PhD
Senior Lecturer in Public Health
School of Medicine,
Medical Sciences and Nutrition
University of Aberdeen
Aberdeen, United Kingdom

David P. Sklar, MD
Professor
College of Health Solutions
Arizona State University
Tempe, Arizona

What is unique to the field of health professions education is the involvement of health professionals crossing disciplinary fields. In this case, the field is social science methodology, crossing into health professions education. This book is about survey research, which is a very common approach in health professions education research. Although it may seem to be a relatively straightforward approach to research and evaluation, many aspects need to be considered. This book is written by authors from the health sciences domain; they know their audience, and they are perfectly able to explain all the methodological issues involved in survey research. Therefore, this text is an easily accessible monograph, providing a systematic overview of what matters in survey research.

The authors have written chapters that follow the various chronological steps in setting up, conducting, analyzing, and reporting survey research. They explain in very accessible language every step, using relevant background from the social science literature. At the same time, the book provides practical suggestions so that readers may make informed decisions and intentional choices. All authors of the book's chapters are experienced researchers, as are its editors. On top of the scientific information, chapters are enriched with "Voice of Experience" sections that provide wisdom from the authors' own survey research experience. These elements lead to a very comprehensive, accessible, and practical overview of survey research. The book is useful for anyone planning survey research in health professions education—not only starting researchers, but also more experienced researchers wanting to check their approach against state-of-the art methodology in survey research. The book is a must-read for anyone involved in survey research.

Cees van der Vleuten, PhD
Professor of Education
Maastricht University, The Netherlands

CONTENTS

Introduction

Andrew W. Phillips, MD, MEd ▪ Steven J. Durning, MD, PhD ▪
Anthony R. Artino, Jr., PhD

Surveys are pervasive in health professions education (HPE), a field that includes physicians, dentists, nurses, physical and occupational therapists, and others. We use surveys to measure learners' opinions about instructors and coursework, to assess trainees' performance of clinical tasks, and to measure everything from attitudes and values to beliefs and behaviors among our research participants. In a study of survey use in HPE research, we found that slightly more than 50% of original research articles in the top three HPE journals employed a survey as part of the methodology.[1] Despite their widespread use, many HPE surveys are poorly constructed and/or inadequately administered. In a follow-up study, we found that 95% of surveys analyzed contained at least one violation of best practices in survey design.[2]

The purpose of this book is twofold: (1) provide essential theory and understanding of methodological concepts necessary to lead high-quality survey studies; and (2) serve as a desk reference for survey guidelines and expert recommendations to help ensure that study methodologies can stand up to rigorous peer reviews. The characteristics that set this book apart from others are its emphasis on the unique audience of health professionals and its concise, practical approach. We provide straightforward examples to illustrate key points in the main text, but also include more intricate examples of real-world difficulties that arise with surveys and propose solutions from experts who have dealt with similar dilemmas personally.

This book is primarily intended for early career educators or researchers in HPE who need a concise explanation and reference for survey methodology, such as those pursuing advanced degrees in HPE (e.g., master's degrees in HPE, master's degrees in education, and doctorates in HPE). It is also designed, by its summaries and checklists, to be a go-to resource for more senior scholars who need a reference to guide their own work, ensuring that all i's are dotted and all t's crossed when designing and conducting a survey study. Thus we will use the general term "survey designers" throughout this book, acknowledging that both educators and researchers are our audience.

A basic understanding of statistical concepts (e.g., t-tests, chi-square, normal distribution, etc.) will help the reader apply the theory and recommendations provided in this book, but it is not required. We refer readers to any number of introductory statistics books, such as Norman and Streiner's *Biostatistics: The Bare Essentials*; Hinkle, Wiersma, and Jurs' *Applied Statistics for the Behavioral Sciences*; or Field's *Discovering Statistics Using IBM SPSS Statistics* (for those who want to learn a data analysis program simultaneously).

The Survey as a Psychometric Instrument

There are many data collection methods that are colloquially referred to as "surveys." However, for the purpose of this book we define **survey** broadly as any instrument comprising prespecified questions (or items) designed to sample and produce statistical information about some aspect(s) of a population.[3,4] We define **questionnaire** as a self-administered survey, regardless of medium. For an instrument to be considered a questionnaire, the requirement is that there is not direct involvement of a survey administrator while the participant is completing the survey.

A properly designed survey can be a solid psychometric instrument, complete with reliability and validity evidence for its intended use. When applicable, survey results can be treated like data from any other assessment or test and can be used to describe anyone within the **sampling frame** (the group of interest being surveyed).

Book Overview

This book provides a six-step, portable method for designing surveys.

Step 1: Needs Assessment is arguably one of the most important steps. This first chapter provides resources to determine whether a survey is the correct methodology, recommends specific places to locate preexisting survey instruments, and explains how to obtain background information necessary to write informed survey questions if there is a need to create a new instrument.

Step 2: Survey Construction applies the theory and evidence, primarily from the cognitive psychology and public opinion polling literature, to help write questions that are clear and likely to be consistently understood by the sampling frame, and thus more likely to hold up to validity testing. This chapter provides the rationale for the best practices for writing items (survey questions).

Step 3: Establishing Evidence provides ample theory to understand our step-by-step instructions to evaluate most survey results for validity and reliability evidence. This chapter describes several schools of thought regarding validity and reliability of evidence.

Step 4: Survey Delivery describes how to increase response rates and makes recommendations about which techniques are most efficient and cost effective.

Step 5: Data Analysis describes how to analyze survey data and interpret findings in the context of the survey instrument as a whole and the specific sampling frame. This chapter also provides relatively straightforward, yet defendable, ways to analyze for nonresponse bias.

Step 6: Reporting Guidelines details how to present findings with an emphasis on how to report findings about individual survey questions (items) and entire surveys in meaningful ways, rather than simply regurgitating scale numbers. In this chapter, we encourage authors to use graphic representations of survey results and describe what was done and what happened in an engaging and persuasive story.

How to Use This Book

We recommend that readers first read the Six Steps above. Note the sequence of steps and the extensive amount of time spent preparing the survey in comparison with actually delivering it. This lopsided balance of time is intentional and will be discussed throughout the book. Then read the book from cover to cover. As readers become more familiar with the concepts, we recommend reading the "Voice of Experience" boxes for practical pearls of wisdom from the authors. From there, we encourage readers to regularly revisit the Six Steps and the associated checklists at the end of each chapter for each survey developed.

Example Case

This book uses one running example through each of the Six Steps to paint a cohesive narrative and hopefully facilitate understanding. We recommend referring back to this case frequently for details.

We are studying the effects of resources for substance abuse among all students at Health Professions Education (HPE) University with a sampling frame of only students who have a history of substance abuse. We solicit responses to a custom questionnaire sent by e-mail and by paper in student mailboxes in the medical school office. The initial information is presented in Table 1.

TABLE 1 ■ Summary of Example Case

Class Characteristics	Total, $N = 400$
Male (%)	200 (50%)
Mean Age	23 years
Academic probation for substance abuse	20 (5%)

Concluding Remarks

We thank the numerous authors for their contributions to make this book possible. We also wish to thank you, the reader, for your education and research contributions. What you do matters, and we hope you find this book to be a useful tool in advancing the field of health professions education.

References

1.   Phillips AW, Friedman BT, Utrankar A, Ta AQ, Reddy ST, Durning SJ. Surveys of health professions trainees: prevalence, response rates, and predictive factors to guide researchers. *Acad Med.* 2017;92(2):222–228. doi:10.1097/ACM. 0000000000001334.
2.   Artino Jr AR, Phillips AW, Utrankar A, Ta AQ, Durning SJ. The questions shape the answers: assessing the quality of published survey instruments in health professions education. *Acad Med.* 2018;93:456–463.
3.   Fowler FJ. *Survey Research Methods.* 5 ed. SAGE Publications; 2013. [eBook].
4.   American Association for Public Opinion Research. Standard definitions: final dispositions of case codes and outcome rates for surveys. https://www.aapor.org/AAPOR_Main/media/publications/Standard-Definitions20169theditionfinal.pdf. Accessed November 25, 2020.

Needs Assessment

Jennifer A. Cleland, PhD ■ Amudha Poobalan, MBBS, PhD ■
Steven J. Durning, MD, PhD

The need for—and difficulty designing—high-quality surveys is one of the main factors that led to the development of this book, and Step 1, the needs assessment, is arguably one of the most important steps in survey methodology. Gillham (2000) pointed out that *"The great popularity with questionnaires is they provide a 'quick fix' for research methodology. No single method has been so abused."* [1]

Here, we discuss the necessary preliminary steps, starting with the definitions of "survey," when and why to use a survey, and drafting the survey objective(s). Next, we discuss gathering supporting information, which includes searching the literature and assessing the stakeholders. Finally, we touch on choosing the survey delivery method and data analyses as they pertain to initial decisions in the survey method process. This chapter also includes tips for synthesizing information from various sources (e.g., literature search, anecdotal evidence, focus groups).

Definition

What is meant by the term "survey method?" *Survey method* can be defined as "the collection of information from a sample of individuals through their responses to questions." [2] For the purposes of this book, and as noted in the book's introduction, a *survey* can be broadly defined as any instrument composed of prespecified questions or *items* designed to sample and produce statistical information about some aspect(s) of a population. [3] A *questionnaire* is a self-administered survey, regardless of medium.

Many texts on survey research design are grounded in the positivistic (scientific) paradigm of objectivity and "one truth." [4] However, the data gathered from survey *items* are often about nonobservable constructs like attitudes, beliefs, and opinions.[5] This can be categorized as descriptive research; some examples are how students rate their own confidence to perform a certain procedure, how trainees rate their learning experience and teachers, and which factors are important in medical student career decision making. In all cases, a survey can provide a point-in-time "snapshot" that is from the perspective of the respondents.[4] Surveys can also be used to explore specific aspects of a situation or to seek explanation and provide data for testing hypotheses.

When and Why to Use a Survey

Surveys are perhaps best used to investigate human phenomena: nonobservable and nonrecorded constructs like attitudes, beliefs, and opinions.[6] A survey is typically not indicated when data are either directly observable or are available via existing sources. For example, daily activity (e.g., amount of time spent exercising) is more accurately recorded by an activity monitor than by a self-reported survey. Likewise, data on student assessments are probably better obtained from centralized records collected in a database rather than by asking individual students to report their grades. Additionally, in most cases, arguably the best time to use a survey is when the focus of the survey (the topic or area) is understood well enough to inform the design of a full range of questions and response options to these questions.[7] If this is not the case, the study should start with some exploratory work to gather information about the topic (e.g., factors influencing medical career preferences); then a questionnaire can be built to explore this in the group of interest (e.g., medical students).

Following on from this, if the primary research question merits the use of a survey, it is quite likely that a similar—if not exactly the same—phenomenon has been surveyed by others. Therefore, if a suitable survey already exists for the purpose of the investigator's query, and that survey was well developed and sufficient validity evidence was gathered for use in a population, then this is usually a contraindication to creating an entirely new survey. This point is discussed in more depth repeatedly in this book. In this chapter, it is assumed that, after a search, no suitable preexisting survey instrument has been identified, meriting the design and development of a new survey. The steps to inform the design and development of a new survey are described in detail later in this chapter and throughout this book.

Draft the Survey Objective(s)

The first step in survey construction is moving from an idea—a question of interest—to survey objective(s), which requires gathering what is already known about the concept and area of interest. The best way to do that is to gather information from the wider literature and relevant people.

Survey objectives inform the research questions and guide the rest of the methodology. Survey objectives are broad, such as "substance abuse among medical students," whereas research questions are narrower, such as "Is there a positive effect from counseling provided to medical students with a history of substance abuse?" Tools like FINER (Feasible, Interesting, Novel, Ethical, and Relevant), used to guide the creation of research questions, are useful for constructing survey objectives as well.

> **VOICE OF EXPERIENCE**
>
> A survey objective is almost never answerable with a single survey question; on the other hand, too often surveys contain a smorgasbord of questions about numerous different topics. Properly addressing an objective requires supporting questions and cohesion of those questions. Limit the number of objectives to adequately answer them.

Gather Supporting Information

The main ways of gathering preliminary information to inform the construction of a survey (i.e., before a single new item is written) are to: 1) carry out a literature review to assess the existing research evidence and the presence of any existing surveys that may inform the new instrument; and 2) collect information from stakeholders to include the opinions of experts in the field and the population that will be sampled. These approaches are discussed later and summarized in Table 2. Gathering this preliminary information will provide a more detailed awareness of the current state of knowledge in the topic area, refine area(s) of interest and a potential sampling frame (who to sample), and clarify the objectives within the broader context.

TABLE 2 ■ Potential Sources of Information to Inform the Construction of a Survey

Source of information	Explanation
Literature review	Review the literature to get ideas about relevant topics from similar studies; use medical databases and educational databases; if there is little information in the health professions education literature, look at the literature from other professions and social sciences.
Existing data	Existing data can inform relevant topics and warrant consideration. This might be existing qualitative data (e.g., semistructured interviews, focus groups) or even anecdotal evidence from committee meetings. It could also be quantitative, such as assessment patterns over time, feedback scores from clinical rotations, etc.
Experience as a practitioner	Personal experience and that of colleagues, plus informal observations, may suggest ideas for question content.
Qualitative data collection	Individual interviews and focus groups.
Consensus process	Qualitative data from meetings and discussions (e.g., individual interviews and focus groups) can inform a formal consensus process (i.e., a Delphi approach). This is a technique whereby a group of experts is encouraged to suggest possible topics/questions, and then gradually adapt these to give rise to a final comprehensive list. The experts may meet as a group, but it is often more common for the exercise to be done in writing (often by email). This level of preplanning is typically only necessary if the survey being developed is for research purposes. The basic steps for conducting a Delphi consensus process[8] are as follows: • Compile a list of questions or statements relating to your research questions, send it to a group of experts, and ask them to respond with their thoughts on the relevance, applicability, and so on. • Produce a group response: Collate the individual responses, organizing them into categories, perhaps noting the frequency or strength of opinion with which topics are suggested. • Send the group response back to individuals for comment; at this stage, the individuals are asked to say how acceptable the group response is to them. Is any disagreement minor or major? • Continue this cycle as necessary, until at some point the greatest extent of agreement has been reached; one or two iterations should be enough.

The importance of gathering this background information cannot be emphasized enough. Building a new instrument without the context of prior, similar work or without input from stakeholders can completely derail a survey because, as a social science tool, the findings from a survey are entirely contextual; that is, they depend on the participants, the setting, the wider context, and other external influences.

The process of developing a new survey is iterative. A loose idea or objective can be refined over time as additional information is gathered from the literature and key stakeholders. Sometimes early ideas and objectives change quite dramatically once more is known about the area of interest; this is typical and to be expected. The key task is to keep the primary (and secondary) objective(s) of the survey in mind when gathering the background information.

Gather Supporting Information: Assess the Literature

LITERATURE REVIEW GOALS

There are three main goals for the literature review: to clearly define the focus of the survey, to position the work within related theory and research in the field (to address knowledge gaps), and to determine whether there are preexisting survey instruments that can be used or adapted for the current purpose[9] (see additional information later in this chapter).

Clarifying the current knowledge base is essential to know which questions are important to ask. For example, in the substance use example from the **Book Introduction**, age should be gathered from participants in the example survey if an association between age and substance abuse was found in prior studies. Current knowledge also establishes constructs of interest. For example, "substance abuse" has many lay definitions but has formal *constructs* that should be used for survey purposes, even surveys not intended for publication.

It is important at this stage to identify the knowledge gaps between the objective(s) of the survey and the sampling frame. For example, there might be prior literature on substance abuse by junior and senior clerkship medical students in other countries but not where HPE University (the fictitious academic center in our running example) is located. The gap is the location.

The third main goal is to identify whether a prior survey instrument that will be appropriate for use or adaptation exists, rather than designing a new survey from scratch. Using an existing tool saves time and, hence, money and, if published, can be used by others to compare findings across studies. Moreover, if a survey designer decides *not* to use an existing, widely accepted tool, it is also necessary to justify that decision. The prior tool may indeed not be appropriate for a given objective, but not using it needs to be justified as much as making a new tool needs to be justified. One important caveat is that many published survey instruments have weak validity and reliability evidence or none at all.[10] Therefore, care should be taken to explore whether and how evidence of validity and reliability was collected for those instrument scores and their intended use (see **Step 3: Establishing Evidence**).

The increased availability of information resources via the Internet can sometimes be a barrier because of the need to filter out peripheral and lower-quality literature. Thus, taking time to develop online search skills will be time well spent. Local medical/university library services are often an underused resource and can support the survey designer. In addition, many online resources provide guidance in searching and evaluating the literature. Box 1 provides guidance for how to systematically assess the literature, from identifying a research question to synthesizing the evidence.

Keeping an open mind and being systematic—methodical, orderly, organized and critical—is appropriate (see Box 1). Choosing the appropriate bibliographical database(s) is also essential to identify the relevant articles. Although some databases focus on articles related to the medical field alone, other databases focus on fields like psychology, sociology, education, and business, to

---

BOX 1 ■ Systematic Steps to a Successful Literature Search

Tips	Example(s)
Literature Search Step 1: Decide on your research question in your own words.	
Make the question as specific as possible	"Which factors influence medical students' specialty choices?"
Literature Search Step 2: Define the terms and concepts.	
Break down the question into keywords, phrases, synonyms, and alternative spellings	"specialty choice" or "career choice"
Use truncation techniques with $ or *	"medic*" or "medic$" (searches "medic," "medicine," "medical education," etc.)
Literature Search Step 3: Use Boolean operators	
Use OR, AND, and NOT	medic$ OR healthcare OR nursing
	medic$ AND student
	medic$ NOT UK
Literature Search Step 4: Limit your search	
Language	English AND French
Publication type	Journal article
Study type	Randomized controlled trial
Year of publication	2010 to present
Stage of training	Medical students
Country of study	United Kingdom
Literature Search Step 5: Select the appropriate database(s)	
Databases vary by timeline and topic	See Table 3 for database examples and details
Literature Search Step 6: Start searching	
Record search terms and results	Use PubMed "save search" feature
	Customize a spreadsheet

---

name just a few (see Table 3). These databases should be reviewed as well, especially if the constructs being measured are topics that might also be relevant elsewhere (e.g., confidence, motivation, and learning strategies).

IDENTIFYING PRIOR SURVEY INSTRUMENTS

A primary goal of the literature search is to look for suitable existing instruments (see Table 4). The outcomes of this search will dictate what the survey designer should do next. In our experience, there are three possible outcomes, each of which has pros and cons.

1) An Ideal Instrument

If an ideal existing tool is found in the literature search, then use it. Be aware that some survey instruments are proprietary, copyrighted, and may require study registration or a fee for use (e.g., the Maslach Burnout Inventory). Many instruments are freely available for use, but permission should nonetheless be sought from the original author. One way to do this is to find the author's e-mail address in the paper or search for the author online, then simply send him or her an e-mail asking for permission with the stipulation of appropriately citing the original work. In our experience, most researchers are delighted if contacted, told a little about the proposed study, and asked for permission to use and cite their survey.

2) The "Nearly But Not Quite Right" Instrument

There is often an existing survey that is nearly but not quite "fit for purpose." Nonetheless, the general tone, number, and organization of the survey *items* may still be relevant. Can the survey be modified to fit the survey designer's needs? Often a good compromise is to create a new instrument

TABLE 3 ■ Popular Bibliographic Databases for Health Professions Education Research

Bibliographic database	Scope of indexing	Pros and Cons
Medline	Compiled by U.S. National Library of Medicine; it focusses on life sciences and biomedical literature	Indexing goes back to 1946 and covers more than 5500 international journals, but more focused on biomedical literature and citations from USA
EMBASE (Experta Medica Database)	Covers biomedical and pharmaceutical literature including drug research, pharmacology, toxicology, drug dependence, etc.	Covers citations from Europe quite widely; indexes more than 3500 international journals and has in-depth indexing (sensitive search)
CINAHL (Cumulative Index to Nursing and Allied Health Literature)	Good resource for allied health discipline subjects such as nursing, alternative and complementary medicine, consumer health, occupational therapy, nutrition, and dietetics	Compiled from National League for Nursing and American Nurses Association; indexing goes from 1982 onward
Cochrane Library	Holds very high-quality literature in interventions field; it indexes interventions in public health, health promotion, surgery, psychology, pharmacology, and healthcare delivery	Covers diagnostic tests as well
ASSIA (Applied Social Sciences Index and Abstracts)	Covers health but also includes literature on economics, politics, race relations and education.	Good source for literature on social science and health
HMIC (Health Management Information Consortium)	Covers literature on health management and policy	Compiled by Information Services of Department of Health; it is a useful resource for healthcare managers and administrators; only United Kingdom based
AMED (Allied and Complementary Medicine Database)	Main focus is on complementary medicine, physiotherapy, occupational therapy, rehabilitation, podiatry, and palliative care	Indexing goes back only to 1985; contains only basic records and covers mainly Europe
ERIC (Education Resources Information Center)	Focus on education literature (not limited to healthcare)	Compiled by Institute of Education Sciences in USA; web based; coverage dates back to 1966; not all peer reviewed
PsychINFO	Covers wide swath of psychology literature	Particularly useful for research on educational psychology and learning theories; indexing is back to the 1800s
Web of Science	Compilation of a variety of databases of variety of disciplines	Includes science, arts, social sciences, medicine fields; indexing is as far back as 1900
Sociological Abstracts	International focus on sociology and behavioral sciences	Good source for interdisciplinary research with social work and social services; reasonable international representation

Note that all of the listed databases except Medline require a subscription to access content. Academic centers generally have subscriptions to at least a few of the mentioned databases.

TABLE 4 ■ Survey and Psychometric Instrument Databases

Database	Notes	Link
American Psychological Association	Commercial online database with thousands of cognitive psychology instruments Commercial books (multiple volumes) of unpublished in primary literature cognitive psychology instruments. Link is for volumes 1–3.	https://www.apa.org/pubs/databases/psyctests/index https://www.apa.org/pubs/books/4316670
Centers for Disease Control and Prevention	Free database with wide range of generic health-related items	https://wwwn.cdc.gov/QBANK/
Buros Center for Testing	Commercial database of instruments for many fields	https://buros.org/mental-measurements-yearbook
EBSCO (Elton B. Stephens Company)	Commercial database of health and social science instruments	https://www.ebsco.com/products/research-databases/health-and-psychosocial-instruments-hapi

but use it alongside one or more published instruments because this allows comparison of proposed work with previous studies plus gives scope to collect data pertinent to the specific research question(s). Keeping the prior instrument intact and adding new, specific *items* helps maintain the strength of the prior instrument. (How to design new questions is covered in the next chapter, **Step 2: Survey Construction.**) Again, copyright issues may be relevant here when using a prior survey.

A word of caution: this might sound contradictory to the previous statement regarding researching existing surveys, but just because a survey has been used in previous studies or published in a peer-reviewed journal does *not* mean it is robust in terms of the validity or reliability evidence of its scores and their intended use. Unfortunately, plenty of low-quality surveys have been published in the medical and HPE literature. For example, one review found that only 6% of patient satisfaction studies used an instrument that had undergone even rudimentary testing,[11] whereas another study found that authors seldom reported anything about validity and reliability evidence in survey-based research studies in HPE.[10] Additionally, even if authors of a published survey have reported extensive validity and reliability evidence in the literature, that does not mean the survey scores will have good reliability or be valid for the new intended use.[12] **Step 3: Establishing Evidence** in this book dives deeply into assessing validity and reliability evidence.

See Box 2 for an abridged quality assurance checklist before using a preexisting survey tool.

BOX 2 ■ Prior Survey Instrument Quality Assurance Checklist

- Were the questions developed on the basis of existing literature?
- Was evidence from the literature supplemented by involvement of experts in the field, colleagues, and members of the target population to ensure validity of the coverage of questions included in the tool (i.e., content validity)?
- Was the survey checked for readability by an appropriate group and modified on the basis of that feedback?
- Did the survey designers ensure respondents could understand and answer the questions on the survey by conducting cognitive interviews (i.e., response process validity)?
- Was the survey pilot tested with an appropriate sample and modified (if applicable) based on results of the pilot test?

3) The Nonexistent Instrument

If there is no appropriate or adaptable preexisting instrument after a well-planned, thorough literature search, a new survey needs to be created from scratch. This is a common situation in HPE. Creating a completely new survey might seem a little intimidating, but, on the other hand, a blank canvas has its benefits in terms of the opportunity to craft a customized instrument that is truly "fit for purpose."

Gather Information: Assess the Stakeholders

IMPORTANCE OF STAKEHOLDERS

After the literature review, the next step is to ascertain whether the survey designer's understanding of a topic of interest matches the ways prospective respondents think about it.[13] If the topic of interest is student satisfaction with anatomy teaching, then insight from students who had recently received anatomy teaching and the staff who designed and delivered the teaching might be particularly valuable. If the topic of interest is which work and nonwork factors are important to residents when considering their first attending (consultant) job options, then perspectives from senior residents and those in the early years of their first attending post are arguably important information.

Talking to stakeholders has many advantages. The selection of *items* and wording (language) of these questions will likely be more informed and in tune with the target group's perceptions. In addition, which *items* are absolutely necessary will likely become apparent after talking with key stakeholders. Surveys should *not* be a chore to complete, and the response rate will be better for a clear and concise survey that uses audience-appropriate language. Through the engagement process, stakeholders may also feel a sense of contribution to the design of the survey. Depending on the method of consultation (see Table 2), they may also understand that their perspective may not be shared by all prospective respondents, and thus there may be a need for compromise. Finally, consulting with people who will be affected by the survey and its results is an example of good research practice. It represents good governance and transparency, demonstrates a desire to engage in meaningful two-way communication, and recognizes the important contribution stakeholders can make to research.

APPROACH TO ASSESSING STAKEHOLDERS

Qualitative methods can be used to collect additional data to refine ideas and find out what others (usually stakeholders) think about the issue at hand. Adding a qualitative stage before writing any items may seem onerous and time consuming, but it does not always have to be extensive. The depth of background work depends on the goals of the survey. If planning a program evaluation, it may be helpful to gather qualitative data relatively informally from the population of interest, such as adding a short discussion of relevant questions to the end of a faculty meeting (which is essentially a focus group) or an e-mail discussion to gather the views and opinions of relevant colleagues. Developing a new survey for publishable research requires more formal qualitative processes, the findings from which may be publishable in their own right and may inform survey development. The objective will inform the approach.

Over the past two or three decades, qualitative research has become a very specialized area, employing a number of rigorous techniques for collecting and analyzing data. For the purposes of this chapter, however, where the main aim of data collection is to inform a survey instrument, a less ambitious, but thorough, approach is usually sufficient. The two methods most commonly used for initial data collection are one-to-one interviews and focus groups (see Table 5).

TABLE 5 ■ **Advantages and Disadvantages of Interviews and Focus Groups**

	Advantages	**Disadvantages**
Interviews	• Good for highly sensitive subjects. • Easier to arrange around participants' schedules, particularly if using video or telephone interviews.	• Can be more vulnerable to interviewer bias than focus groups. • Time consuming.
Focus Groups	• May facilitate discussions around areas of shared interest. • Less time consuming and expensive than interviews.	• Can be difficult to convene when potential participants are geographically distant from one another or when they have busy schedules (e.g., health professionals). • Need skillful facilitation so participants discuss topics, not just respond individually to the facilitator's questions. • Need to manage the discussions so participants do not talk over one another.

Discussions in both interviews and focus groups are usually guided by a semistructured topic guide consisting of headings that describe the main areas to be explored and a few prompts to stimulate the conversation if needed. The literature review, together with informal discussions with relevant stakeholders and experts, will provide guidance on which topics are likely to be relevant to the proposed research and/or quality assurance project. Conversation points in both interviews and focus groups often change over time as topics are better understood; it is a normal part of the process.

Data collection will be optimized when participants feel at ease, and, to this end, attention to detail when organizing meetings with investigators should be a priority. The date, time, and location of meetings should be convenient for participants and, when possible, expenses (e.g., travel costs) covered. Meeting rooms should be comfortable, away from potential interruptions, and refreshments (e.g., water) should be provided. Participants should be reminded that information shared with the survey designers will be treated as confidential. Additionally, focus groups should be guided by "rules," set out at the start, impressing on participants the importance of respecting the views of others and the need for confidentiality.

 VOICE OF EXPERIENCE

It is ideal to audio record the interviews (with the permission of participants) for later transcription. This practice minimizes the chance of missing important points being made and allows the facilitator to concentrate on the speaker and the flow of conversation, rather than recording data in handwritten notes. Audio recordings can then be transcribed in a word processing package for later analysis. A little paranoia is not a bad thing here: make two recordings, so you have one as backup!

The sample to be included in these qualitative exercises should include a range of perspectives. *Sampling frames* might include employment groups (e.g., consultants), student groups (e.g., first-year medical students), organization lists (e.g., members of a professional organization), or publicly available lists (e.g., homes in a particular district).

Purposive sampling (in which survey designers intentionally select participants based on specific characteristics such as age, positions held, or expertise) is ideal for the qualitative part of gathering background information because it aims to ensure representation from a range of characteristics that are relevant to the research question. *Snowball sampling* (in which those already participating in the study are asked to identify others who might be willing to participate) is helpful when recruiting is otherwise difficult. Neither group is meant to be a sample for inferential statistics, but rather a small, broadly representative group of experts and stakeholders—a completely different goal from distribution of the final survey instrument.

There is no fixed, ideal number of participants for focus groups and interviews that inform survey creation. However, factors to consider when setting a target sample size include:

- Stakeholders: Who are the people most involved with or affected by the topic of the research? Should different subgroups be represented as stakeholders?
- Participant characteristics: Are data from a range of ages, ethnicities, genders, geographical locations of interest, etc.?
- Resources: How much time has been allocated to data collection, and how much money will be available to spend on survey team salaries, travel, participant expenses, room rental (hire), or transcribing costs, etc.?
- Data saturation: At what point does little or no new data emerge from subsequent interviews? This factor will only become clear as interviews progress.

For the purpose of survey development, a fairly straightforward thematic analysis will typically be sufficient.[14] The main aim of thematic qualitative analysis is to reduce raw data, which is usually voluminous and diverse, to meaningful summaries; themes and subthemes are identified from the data that concisely encapsulate participants' views and experiences. See **Step 5: Data Analysis** for more comprehensive analysis guidance, although that is rarely needed at this point.

ETHICS PERMISSION

Remember that it is important to obtain permission from the relevant ethical bodies in any data collection exercise for research purposes (see Table 6). Participants must also grant their informed consent for any formal qualitative data collection. Sometimes, a survey designer applies for ethical approval for the qualitative stage of data collection (survey construction) separately from the ethical approval for final survey administration. Always check with the ethics office of the institution where the project is being conducted for any questions.

TABLE 6 ■ **Is Ethics Permission Required?**

Objective	Guidance
Internal program Curriculum evaluation Audit	Formal ethical approval probably not required, but conduct data collection in an ethical manner (e.g., make clear that taking part is voluntary; do not coerce participants).
Research that will be published or discussed in a public forum	A formal application for ethical approval from a particular research ethics committee is probably required, depending on the context. Many studies will be exempted, but obtaining formal exemption is required in most countries. • Survey of medical students may require approval from a university ethics board and, in some cases, additional approval from the dean of the medical school. • Survey of residents, colleagues, or patients may require approval from a clinical/healthcare ethics board and, in some cases, additional approval from relevant residency program authorities.

Choosing the Delivery Method

Surveys can be administered by mail, phone, in-person, or online, and there are different considerations for each delivery modality. **Step 4: Survey Delivery** is dedicated to survey delivery. The current chapter focuses on decision making regarding the best format of a survey for the objective(s) and to inform the next step, **Step 2: Survey Construction,** which varies with delivery method. Each mode of administration has pros and cons. For example, if an interviewer is asking the questions, think about how they will sound, especially if they are sensitive questions like the substance abuse example (see **Book Introduction**). If the objective requires visual aids such as graphs or medical images, think about which modalities can include images.

The best approach will also depend on the research question, existing knowledge, and practical factors such as time, resources, and available staff. Is there a full-time researcher or staff member working on the project who is trained in telephone interviewing, or is this a single-person project alongside many other tasks? If the latter, then face-to-face/personal methods of survey data collection may not be feasible. It is helpful to read **Step 4: Survey Delivery** before making final delivery choices. It is mentioned here as a reminder to consider delivery method practicalities up front.

VOICE OF EXPERIENCE

Preexisting knowledge of the population of interest is useful in deciding the mode of administration. For example, one of us (JC) had a research question directed at final-year students across the five Scottish medical schools. Historically, response rates for surveys distributed by e-mail were low for this population, so JC contacted the medical program leaders at each school and asked if they would support their students taking part in the study. After obtaining the necessary ethical permissions, study information was e-mailed by the respective institutions to their students, and JC was given a timetable slot at each medical school to present the study and invite the final-year students to complete the survey. This face-to-face and paper-and-pencil administration was time consuming but resulted in a response rate more than 80%.[15,16]

Data Analyses

The last part of preparation before embarking on writing questions is to consider the planned analyses. There should be a plan up front for which variables will be measured and how they will be measured; these both, of course, influence question writing but depend on the study objectives. For example, is it most important to know if the respondents *ever* used illicit substances (a dichotomous answer of yes or no) or how frequently they used illicit substances during a confined period of time (an integer answer)? Similar to the decision on survey delivery, it is a good idea to read **Step 5: Data Analysis** prior to writing any questions, and it is mentioned here as a reminder to consider analyses early. Appendix 1 is a basic example worksheet to help the novice survey designer plan a survey.

Needs Assessment Checklist

- ☐ Determine survey objective(s) (iterative process).
- ☐ Define sampling frame (iterative process).
- ☐ Determine whether survey is the best method to achieve the objective(s).
- ☐ Obtain ethics permission (as applicable).
- ☐ Assess the literature.
  - ☐ Iterative search process
  - ☐ Relevant databases
  - ☐ Prior survey instruments and their quality
- ☐ Assess the stakeholders.
  - ☐ All parties that affect or are affected by the objective(s)
  - ☐ Informal vs. formal assessment to inform survey development
    - ☐ Experience/observation
    - ☐ Focus groups and/or interviews
    - ☐ Consensus approaches.
- ☐ Consider logistical and financial factors that influence delivery method(s).
- ☐ Consider planned analyses to inform how items are written.

References

1. Gillham B. *Developing a Questionnaire*. London: Continuum; 2000:123.
2. Check J, Schutt RK. *Research Methods in Education*. Thousand Oaks, CA: Sage; 2012:160.
3. Fowler FJ. *Improving Survey Questions: Design and Evaluation. Applied Social Research Methods Series* Improving Survey Questions: Design and Evaluation. Applied Social Research Methods Series, Vol. 38 Thousand Oaks, CA: Sage Publishing; 1995.
4. Cleland JA. Exploring versus measuring: considering the fundamental differences between qualitative and quantitative research. In: Cleland JA, Durning SJ, eds. *Researching Medical Education*. Oxford: Wiley; 2015:3–14.
5. Singleton RA, Straits BC. *Approaches to Social Research*. New York: Oxford University Press; 2009.
6. Artino Jr AR, La Rochelle JS, Dezee KJ, Gehlbach H. Developing questionnaires for educational research: AMEE Guide No. 87. *Med Teach*. 2014;36(6):463–474.
7. Phillips AW. Proper Application of Surveys as a Study Methodology. *West J EM*. 2017;18(1):8–11.
8. Hsu CC, Sandford BA. The Delphi technique: making sense of consensus. Practical assess. *Res & Eval*. 2017;12:10.
9. Gehlbach H, Artino AR, Durning SJ. AM last page: survey development guidance for medical education researchers. *Acad Med 2010*. 2010;85:925.
10. Artino AR, Phillips AW, Utrankar A, Ta AQ, Durning SJ. The questions shape the answers: assessing the quality of published survey instruments in health professions education. *Acad Med*. 2018;93:456–463.
11. Sitzia J. How valid and reliable are patient satisfaction data? An analysis of 195 studies. *Int J Quul Health Care*. 1999;11:319–328.
12. Phillips AW, Diller D, Williams S, Park YS, Fisher J, Biese K, et al. The Council of Emergency Medicine Residency Directors Speaker Evaluation Form for Medical Conference Planners. *AEM Educ Train*. 2017;1(4):340–345.
13. Gehlbach H, Brinkworth ME. Measure twice, cut down error: a process for enhancing the validity of survey scales. *Rev Gen Psychol*. 2011;15:380–387.
14. Saldana J. *The Coding Manual for Qualitative Researchers*. 2 ed. Los Angeles: Sage; 2013.
15. Cleland JA, Johnston P, Watson V, Krucien N, Skatun D. What do UK medical students value most in their career? A discrete choice experiment. *Med Educ*. 2017;51:839–851.
16. Van Geest JB, Johnson TP, Welch VL. Methodologies for improving response rates in surveys of physicians: a systematic review. *Eval Health Prof*. 2007;30:303–321.

Further Reading

Gillham B. *Developing a Questionnaire (Real World Research)*. London: Continuum; 2000. *Self-explanatory.*

Boynton PM, Greenhalgh T. Selecting, designing, and developing your questionnaire. *BMJ*. 2004;328(7451):1312–1315. *An overview.*

Converse JM, Presser S. *Survey Questions: Handcrafting the Standardized Questionnaire*. Sage University Paper series on Quantitative Applications in the Social Sciences, No. 07-063. Thousand Oaks, CA; SAGE: 1986. *A good succinct introduction.*

Fowler FJ Jr. *Improving Survey Questions: Design and Evaluation, Applied Social Research Methods Series* (Vol 38). Thousand Oaks, CA; SAGE Publications: 1995. *A good introductory text*

Ritchie J, Lewis J (Eds). *Qualitative Research Practice. A Guide for Social Science Students and Researchers*. London; Sage; 2003. *A classic guide.*

Survey Construction

Jeffrey LaRochelle, MD, MPH ■ Anthony R. Artino, Jr., PhD

Having accomplished the primary task of defining the specific questions to be asked or constructs to be measured, the next step focuses on writing and testing the actual items that will populate the survey. Therefore this chapter focuses on helping survey designers (researchers and educators) write high-quality items that are interpreted consistently by every respondent and in the way the item writer intended. Before describing the "nuts and bolts" of item writing, there is some benefit in reviewing a bit of cognitive psychology to better understand how respondents approach, understand, and answer survey items. This is important because a large proportion of the error associated with surveys is derived from problems that occur when respondents have trouble making sense of the questions being asked, which, in turn, makes it difficult to generate meaningful answers.[1]

The chapter begins with a brief overview of how respondents think about and answer survey items. Next, the chapter covers the three main steps required to create a new survey: 1) writing items, 2) visually displaying items, and 3) testing items.

How Respondents Answer Survey Items

COGNITIVE RESPONSE PROCESS MODEL

Several models describe the underlying cognitive functions associated with answering items on a survey, but the *cognitive response process model* (see Fig. 1) outlined in the early 1980s has stood the test of time and provides a relatively simple framework for understanding these complex processes.[2] There are four basic processes outlined in the response process model: 1) item comprehension;

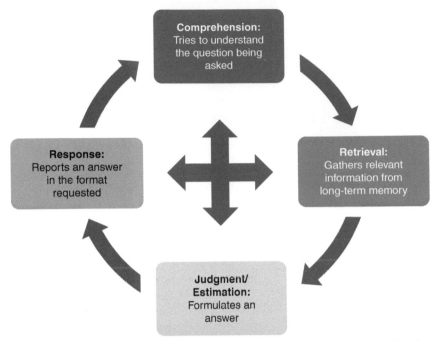

Fig. 1 Cognitive Response Process Model. Note that movement between the processes is neither linear nor unidirectional.

2) data retrieval; 3) data integration into a judgment or estimation; and 4) response reporting. Although the model suggests a natural order from comprehension to reporting, in practice, respondents often jump around, cycling back and forth between processes while reading and answering items. Using the example survey on substance abuse from the **Book Introduction** as an illustration: After comprehending a question about the frequency of Alcoholics Anonymous attendance, a respondent might begin searching his or her long-term memory (retrieval) and counting or estimating the visits (judgment/estimation). However, after several seconds of mental math, the respondent might wonder, "Wait, this is a large number; this can't be what the question is really asking, can it?" At which point, the respondent might jump back and reread the question to ensure he or she understands it correctly (comprehension).

With this processing model as a backdrop, one of the main goals for a survey designer is to write items that every respondent understands in the same way. Moreover, the item should be understood in the way the item was intended to be understood by the survey designer. To be sure, respondents will have different answers for the questions being asked; after all, that is the whole point of collecting data using a survey. However, the way the item is *understood* should not vary from respondent to respondent. Therefore it is unsurprising that problems with item comprehension are some of the most common causes of survey error.[3] It is also why this component of the processing model should be an area of focus for survey designers.

Item Comprehension

There are three main ways respondents can miscomprehend an item. The first involves ambiguity in the syntax of the item and relates to differences in meaning based on item phrasing. Consider the item:

The poodle has 5 puppies. The collie has 7 puppies.
How many more puppies does the collie have?

Many respondents will give the correct answer, "2"; however, some respondents may answer "None." Despite the seemingly simple nature of this example, ambiguity arises from the syntax of the question: Is this item asking how many more puppies the collie has in comparison with the poodle, or is it asking if the collie had any more (additional) puppies? Interpreting the item in the latter way leads to the erroneous answer: "None."

The second problem arises from potential ambiguity in the meaning of specific words or phrases. For example, consider the question:

How many assessments have you given your students this semester?

Again, this is a seemingly simple question, but respondents may have different interpretations of the word "assessments" and therefore not know which assessments to count. For example, should formative assessments given during class be counted? What about assessments that ask students to evaluate their own knowledge (i.e., self-assessments). If there is a pretest at the beginning of class and a corresponding posttest at the end, are these counted as one or two assessments? Does the module assessment given by all the module teachers count as an assessment "you" have given? In this case, the definition of a fairly simple word like "assessments" can be understood in any number of different ways.

Finally, respondents will often make assumptions about the intent of an item based on personal or contextual information. For example, an item previously answered on a survey may have asked a respondent about his or her participation in team sports during medical school. Based on this item, the respondent may assume a subsequent question about participation in physical activity should exclude team sports because the survey already asked about this. Alternatively, a respondent might only consider physical activity that took place as part of team activities, excluding other types of physical activity. Even clearly written items are susceptible to such comprehension errors. Fortunately, several principles can be used to improve both item clarity and comprehension, and there are ways to pretest items to facilitate clarity. These are discussed later in the chapter.

Data Retrieval

Regardless of how respondents interpret a particular item, another necessary step in the cognitive response model is the retrieval of appropriate data from their long-term memory needed to answer the question. Recall bias is a long-recognized area of concern for survey developers, but some specific aspects of the retrieval process are worth discussing in more detail. Retrieval is the process of moving information from long-term memory into working memory. Although a great deal of information can be stored in long-term memory, the way in which a respondent has coded that information will often dictate how easily that information can be retrieved.[1] For example, many respondents will be able to recall detailed memories about where they were or what they were doing on September 11, 2001 (the day two airplanes hit the World Trade Center in New York City); however, they may not be able to recall any of that same information about a random day in August 2001. This example further illustrates the importance of understanding the audience, because 9/11 will likely be far more memorable for citizens of the United States than for citizens of other countries. The way in which an item triggers (or fails to trigger) a memory will influence retrieval and, ultimately, how a respondent answers the item. Difficulties in retrieval of information from long-term memory can lead to both overreporting and underreporting events, which can lead to unwanted variance (i.e., errors) in survey responses. Providing historical cues in the form of major life events (e.g., anniversaries, graduations, etc.) may improve the accuracy of retrieval.[1]

Data Integration Into a Judgment or Estimate

Once a respondent has retrieved the appropriate information to answer an item, that information must be synthesized to form a judgment or an estimate. Respondents use a variety of strategies to construct a particular judgment or estimate, and each strategy can introduce errors and unwanted variation in responses.[4] Respondents may use a relatively labor-intensive, thoughtful process of recalling memories of specific events to formulate a judgment based on those memories, or they may use a less labor-intensive process of recalling general information about a particular memory to formulate a judgment based on an extrapolation of that information. This is reflective of the classic system 1 (fast, low effort, and relatively unconscious decisions) and system 2 (slow, higher effort, and more methodical decisions) decision making.

Respondents will preferentially use the less effortful system 1 processes unless they understand that the effort to engage in a more laborious approach (system 2) is worthwhile. In general, system 1 decision making can be prone to a variety of heuristic biases. For example, availability bias may lead to an overestimation in the frequency of a rare event, or representative bias may lead to an inaccurate categorization of an item if it fits a particular prototypical representation in the mind of the respondent. Judgment formulation may be influenced by a variety of factors in the survey itself to include the relative importance of a particular item or how the respondent has answered previous items on the survey.[5,6] Previous items may activate memories and/or judgments that will influence judgments on future items. And so, the order in which a survey presents items can have important impacts on the responses and outcomes (and thus must be considered by survey designers).

➡ VOICE OF EXPERIENCE

In a way, the items on a survey can be thought of as "mini interventions" that can have an effect on answers (responses) to items presented later in the survey. The challenge is knowing ahead of time how a given item might affect respondents' answers on later items. The best way to deal with this challenge is to thoroughly pretest the entire survey using techniques such as expert reviews and cognitive interviews (see later sections of this chapter).

➡ VOICE OF EXPERIENCE

In a study of worksite health promotion program participants, an anonymous survey of participants about their weekly program adherence and goal achievement obtained different results depending on the question wording: "How often did you lie in your weekly goal report?" versus "How truthful were you in your weekly goal report?" Perhaps unsurprisingly, few participants were willing to acknowledge lying, but most were willing to report that they were less than 100% truthful.[4] Using less-threatening language can reduce missing data and improve overall response rates.

Response Reporting

Finally, respondents must generate an answer to the survey item that most closely matches the judgment or estimate they have constructed. Although some survey items allow for open-ended answers (e.g., comment boxes), items often have a defined set of closed-ended answer choices in the form of categorical, ordinal, Likert-type, or other similar response options. Within that framework, respondents must find an answer category that most closely matches their judgment or estimate. Respondents may use examples from their experiences to establish the extremes for a set of response options and thereby compare and contrast their judgments using those examples as a general guide.[1] Therefore, it is important to provide response options that closely approximate the judgments that respondents may determine on their own for each item. Regardless, it is important to remember that unwanted variance may arise from a respondent's preference (or aversion) to select answers at the extremes of the response scale. For example, respondents often give more attention to response options that are listed at the beginning of a vertically oriented written list, which can lead to *primacy effects* (i.e., respondents being more likely to select those initial items in the list rather than later items). On the other hand, on survey items presented verbally (as in a phone interview), respondents tend to favor response options said last, leading to *recency effects*.[7,8] There may also be social biases associated with overreporting of socially desirable behaviors and underreporting of socially undesirable behaviors, such as in the example survey on substance abuse (see **Book Introduction**).

OPTIMIZATION AND SATISFICING

Respondents engage with the cognitive processes described earlier to varying degrees (if at all) based on their motivation to respond, which is strongly influenced by characteristics of the survey and the context in which it is being administered. *Optimization* occurs when respondents are fully engaging in all four of the cognitive processes; i.e., they are being thoughtful, working their way through all four cognitive processes. On the other hand, *satisficing* occurs when respondents have become relatively disengaged with the survey and begin taking shortcuts to conserve mental energy. This circumstance often occurs when the effort of answering the entire survey, or even a particular survey item, outweighs the motivation to respond accurately and completely.[9] Moreover, the motivation to provide thoughtful and complete responses may wax and wane during the completion of a given survey, and motivation can even be thwarted completely when a respondent encounters a particularly confusing or poorly written item. The best way to discourage respondents from satisficing is to avoid poorly written and poorly formatted items (see Table 7) and to pretest the survey before use.

TABLE 7 ■ Survey Respondent Cognitive Pitfalls and Their Design Solutions

Cognitive Process	Problems	Solutions
Comprehension	Phrasing	• Avoid double-barreled items. • Use positive language. • Avoid reverse coded items. • Use the active voice.
	Definition	• Define terms and phrases. • Understand the audience. • Match vocabulary by education, age, ethnicity, etc.
	Intent	• Understand the audience. • Be aware of ordering effects.

Retrieval	Recall Bias	• Provide historical cues.
		  • Personal (anniversary, birthday, graduation, etc.)
		  • World events (Olympics, elections, etc.)

Judgment/ Estimation	Availability Bias	• Provide a framework to assist with estimations.
	Representativeness Bias	• Avoid reliance on prototypical presentations.
	Ordering effect	• Consider different versions of the survey. • Pretest to look for ordering effects.
Reporting	Primacy	• Provide verbal labels. • Ensure options are visually balanced.
	Recency	• Place response options in single row or column (not both). • Use "forced-choice" (Yes/No) response options as opposed to "Check all that apply."
	Mismatch	• Avoid agree/disagree response options. • Ensure response options match item stems. • Use an appropriate number of response options (5–7 options are typically sufficient for Likert-type response options). • Avoid overlapping and nonmutually exclusive response options.

VOICE OF EXPERIENCE

Respondents can easily become demotivated and begin satisficing—i.e., being less thoughtful and complete—while working through a survey. The best defense against satisficing is to create a high-quality survey that follows evidence-informed best practices and then evaluate that survey using pretesting techniques.

Writing Survey Items

There is a science to writing good survey items; that said, there is also a fair amount of art as well (as with most things in the social sciences). The process is iterative and, just like the cognitive process model, is not typically done in a linear fashion in the real world. Certain fundamental decisions should be made for almost all surveys, and those decisions can (and often do) change as the instrument is tested. Some of these decisions are presented in this section, summarized in Box 3, and listed in a more detailed survey design checklist in Appendix 2. The next section is likely oversimplified and does not represent every possible design consideration for every survey, but it is meant to give the novice survey designer a place to start. It is by no means the only way to approach item writing. Most of the decisions in this section are meant for closed-ended items, with an additional subsection at the end dedicated to open-ended items.

BOX 3 ■ Fundamental Considerations for Item Writing

Note that these considerations can be addressed in any order and are interconnected.
- Appropriate language for sampling frame
- Question vs. statement stem
- Response option types
- Number of response options
- Nonsubstantive response options (e.g., N/A, no opinion)
- Item polarity (i.e., unipolar vs. bipolar)
- Open-ended items

VOICE OF EXPERIENCE

Sometimes it is particularly difficult to determine the best way to present an item. If this occurs, write that same item in different ways and test various options in cognitive interviewing before the rest of the instrument is tested. It is better to test the item up front rather than struggle with it during later testing or analysis.

APPROPRIATE LANGUAGE FOR SAMPLING FRAME

One of the first considerations in writing survey items is to clearly define the target audience. This clear definition often includes educational background and primary language, but it should also take into account a variety of demographic information such as ethnicity, age, place of residence (both regional and/or urban, rural, etc.), and occupation, among others. Although some surveys may be designed to cross over many of these defining features, each factor can potentially influence the way in which respondents understand the items on a survey. Once the target audience is defined, the next challenge is to write items using the vocabulary of the target audience and in a way that will promote clear and consistent comprehension of those items. (Using medical terminology is a common challenge in health professions education [HPE] research, especially when knowledge may vary, such as with students who likely have different knowledge bases.) To address potential errors in comprehension that can arise because of ambiguity in item vocabulary, survey designers should consider providing definitions for terms that could be confusing.[10,11] These definitions can be in an opening statement followed by a series of items, or they can be parenthetically embedded in the actual item stem itself. The key feature is providing a clear definition of ambiguous terms or phrases that is easily accessible and in close proximity to the item.

QUESTION VS. STATEMENT STEM

At its core, a survey is a kind of conversation between the survey designer and the respondents. Therefore it is important to develop items in a way that mirrors a conversation, by asking clear questions and avoiding unnecessarily confusing language. The use of statements with agree/disagree response options is one of the most common decisions that breaks the conversation premise. Many experts would deem the use of agree/disagree items as a common mistake made by survey writers; as such, it has been repeatedly identified as a suboptimal format for item design.[9,12-14] For example, when conversing with another person, very seldom do individuals list a bunch of statements and then ask the other person to rate the extent to which they agree or disagree with the statements. It is just not a typical way that people talk, and numerous studies have demonstrated that this type of format is not ideal for surveys either. In particular, such an approach has been found to increase satisficing and ambiguity and diminish the quality of the responses obtained.[15,16] In an extensive study involving participants across 14 countries in Europe, the authors found that item-specific response options resulted in scores with significantly better reliability and validity than agree/disagree response options did for the same items.[16] Furthermore, agree/disagree response options often confound the construct being measured with the degree to which the respondent is agreeable (note: agreeableness is one of the Big Five personality traits).[17] Thus, using agree/disagree response options may encourage acquiescence on the part of respondents, thereby failing to capture the construct being assessed in a meaningful way, be that an opinion, an attitude, or a belief.[18]

Finally, agree/disagree response options may also promote snap judgments, leading to an abbreviated or incomplete retrieval and synthesis of memory that could further erode the accuracy of responses.[9] Because a survey is essentially a conversation, it is better to avoid statements and agree/disagree response options and instead write items as questions with construct-specific response options. Doing so makes the survey more conversational and encourages respondents to process the survey items as if being engaged in a conversation.[19] In short, the use of construct-specific response options in combination with questions instead of statements is an evidence-informed method for not only reinforcing the intent of the item, but also reducing the cognitive burden for respondents.[15]

RESPONSE OPTION TYPES

Items with closed-ended response options may have a variety of formats, including nominal options, dichotomous options, ordinal options, Likert-type options, and ranking options (these are described below in items a through d). Although Likert-type options are quite common, they may not be the best format for every item. Rather, the response option format that a survey designer selects should first and foremost match the purpose of the item and the intended approach to analyzing the item.

    a. *Nominal Options.* Nominal options are useful when no hierarchal relationship exists between the options; that is, the options do not have any implicit numeric value (e.g., gender, city of origin, etc.). Items with nominal response options should allow only one choice to be selected. Nominal options create data that are typically analyzed using nonparametric inferential statistical tests.

b. *Dichotomous Options.* If the options that characterize an item are truly dichotomous (e.g., yes/no), then designers should provide that type of response option. Similarly, the response options should be binary if the planned analysis makes the most sense with an item that is binary. For example, substance use can be viewed as frequency (integer number) or dichotomy (use vs. abstinence). The "correct" item design depends on what the survey designer is trying to convey and the intended approach for data analysis.

c. *Likert-Type Options.* In general, Likert-type options are useful to inform about frequency (e.g., how often), comparisons (e.g., how important), personal attributes (e.g., how confident), etc. In the strictest definition, a *Likert item* (as opposed to a Likert-type item) uses agree/disagree response options, which, as described earlier, are not ideal for surveys. Instead, a better approach is to match the information being requested by the item to the response options. In other words, if a designer is seeking to understand how confident a learner is in reading an ECG, then the item should use response options that ask about level of confidence (e.g., not at all confident, somewhat confident, etc.). Appendix 3 provides a sampling of common Likert-type response options.

d. *Ranking.* Ranking can be helpful when designers want to directly compare a group of (usually) desirable options, such as, "Rank your favorite residency-sponsored wellness events." The options are a specific and defined set (either it was a sponsored wellness event, or it wasn't), and they are all about a single item of interest, the favorite wellness event. It is worth noting that the same information can be gained by asking respondents to rate a number of response options using a common, Likert-type scale. The rating approach allows for different items to receive the same rating and still allows the item scores to be rank ordered after the fact. Both rating and ranking are reasonable approaches, but the survey designer should carefully match the format chosen to the intent of the question. Consider this example:

Rank the following items in order of personal importance, where 1 is "most important" and 6 is "least important":

Family
Health
Money
Career
Freedom
Happiness

In this case where all of the options might be considered quite important, a *ranking* task might make the most sense because it forces respondents to make difficult choices among options that are all desirable. On the other hand, because the order of each item on a ranked list depends on all other items (i.e., they are not "independent observations"), ranking tasks can be cognitively challenging for respondents, especially ranking tasks that have more than about five or six items. Thus for long lists, it often makes more sense to ask respondents to rate each item (e.g., on a scale from 1 to 5, where 1 is "not at all important" and 5 is "extremely important"). Respondents can complete this type of rating task quite easily, and the survey designer can still rank-order the mean ratings for each item after all respondents have answered. Notably, asking respondents to directly rank options generally results in stronger reliability and validity outcomes in comparison with having them rate individual items and then comparing the individual means.[8,20,21] Ultimately, the choice between rating vs. ranking depends on a number of factors (e.g., the purpose of the survey item, the number of items on the list, the education level of the respondents, etc.). Therefore survey designers are encouraged to consider these factors and make thoughtful, deliberate choices. The dilemma also represents another good example of why pretesting survey items is so important.

NUMBER OF RESPONSE OPTIONS

An issue that many survey designers agonize over relates to the question of the total number of response options and whether to use an odd or even number of options. Odd numbers typically allow for a middle response, often a "neutral" response, for items that use bipolar response options (see discussion on item polarity later in this chapter), whereas even numbers do not. If the answer to an item truly has a middle or "neutral" response, then forcing respondents to "pick a side" by using an even number of response options may not be a good approach because it increases item difficulty and may decrease respondent motivation. Decreased respondent motivation means more *satisficing* and, ultimately, lower-quality responses. On the other hand, providing a neutral response when not necessary may present an opportunity to quickly satisfice and thus results in less accurate data. Our recommended approach is to include a middle or neutral option if and when it is a potentially meaningful response. For example, the middle option of "just the right amount of time" is meaningful for an item that asks, "Was the class period too long, just the right amount of time, or too short?"

VOICE OF EXPERIENCE

Although strong opinions exist on either side of the odd or even response option debate, whether or not a midpoint is offered has very little effect on the resulting quality of the data or conclusions that can be drawn.[22,23]

In addition to odd or even, the question of how many options to supply often challenges designers. On the one hand, providing too few response options may impair a respondent's ability to appropriately map his or her judgments to the survey (i.e., there simply are not enough points for the respondent to accurately reflect his or her opinion). On the other hand, providing too many response options can also be problematic: a 100-point response scale may seem intuitively obvious to the survey designer, but the respondents may not be able to make such fine-grain distinctions. Although the literature varies regarding the "optimal number" of response options to include, several scholars have suggested that the optimal number likely lies somewhere between 4 and 9 response options, although 5 to 7 response options is typically sufficient.[15,24,25]

VOICE OF EXPERIENCE

If it is proving difficult to think of labels for all the response options, it might be a sign that there are too many options. Similarly, if there are more meaningful labels than the number of options planned, it might be a sign that the number of options needs to be expanded. Let the expected range of answers drive the size of the response scale, not a predetermined "best" number.

NONSUBSTANTIVE RESPONSE OPTIONS

Along with number of response options, a common question is whether to include a "not applicable," "no opinion," or "don't know" option. Such categories are often referred to as nonsubstantive response options because they are not really part of the continuum of the other Likert-type options (i.e., they are not a functional part of the construct being measured). Unless the answer might reasonably be "not applicable" (e.g., number of prior pregnancies if the respondent is male) or "don't know" for an item that is asking for factual information that someone might not know (e.g., "What was your SAT score?" 30 years after the exam), then survey designers should avoid such nonsubstantive response options. The primary rationale for avoiding such options, from a design standpoint, is that they allow respondents to sidestep the work of giving a response even when they actually have an opinion or know the answer.[22] Where possible, survey designers should not use nonsubstantive options because an "N/A" or "no opinion" or "don't know" response is essentially a nonresponse, and item nonresponse subtracts from the higher response rates survey designers seek.

 VOICE OF EXPERIENCE

In general, nonsubstantive response options should be avoided. However, there are times when they might be appropriate. When trying to decide, for example, whether a "no opinion" option might be appropriate, survey designers should ask themselves, "Can respondents reasonably provide an educated guess to this question?" If the answer is, "Yes," then the nonsubstantive response option should not be used.

ITEM POLARITY

Another common question is the choice between the use of bipolar response options and unipolar options. Bipolar options progress from negative to positive and may have a neutral point in the middle (e.g., completely dissatisfied, somewhat dissatisfied, neutral, somewhat satisfied, completely satisfied). Unipolar options, on the other hand, range from zero to some finite or infinite value (e.g., never, rarely, sometimes, often, always). For certain constructs, like frequency, the only option is unipolar because respondents cannot do something for a negative amount of time. But for other constructs, like satisfaction or motivation, the choice between unipolar and bipolar may require a bit more thought. For instance, when asking medical students how satisfied they are with a course, they can be asked this question in at least two different ways, as demonstrated in the examples in Fig. 2. The choice of which to use is really up to the survey designer and should relate to the purpose of the survey and its intended use.

Unipolar version: How satisfied were you with today's class?

not at all satisfied	somewhat satisfied	moderately satisfied	quite satisfied	extremely satisfied

Bipolar version: How satisfied or dissatisfied were you with today's class?

very dissatisfied	slightly dissatisfied	neither satisfied nor dissatisfied	slightly satisfied	very satisfied

Fig. 2 Examples of Bipolar and Unipolar Items. In this example, note that the wording of the question stem aligns with the response options. In the unipolar version, the question asks only about satisfaction, and the response options range from zero satisfaction to extreme satisfaction. In the bipolar version, the question asks about satisfaction or dissatisfaction, and the options range from negative (very dissatisfied) to positive (very satisfied). The key point is to ensure parallelism between the question stem and the response options being used. If the stem suggests a bipolar answer, then both the positive and negative sides of the issue should be stated in the stem.

OPEN-ENDED ITEMS

A critical step in item writing is to create a set of response options that will match the intended meaning of the item. Although many surveys are designed with closed-ended response options, certain items may require an open-ended option, or the entire item may need to be open-ended.

For example, if the universe of possible or likely responses is not well known by the survey designer, then an open-ended item might be better, allowing respondents to provide more complete and potentially more accurate information. However, it is important to note that responses to open-ended items can still be influenced by characteristics of the item itself, such as how much space is provided for the answer. All else being equal, if a survey designer provides a small answer space for a given open-ended item, respondents will be more likely to provide a short answer consistent with the space provided.[26–29]

Providing an "Other" option (often combined with a comment box) alongside closed-ended response options can be a potentially valuable source of data if a set of likely or probable responses is anticipated, but not all possibilities are clearly defined (e.g., gender). This option can provide respondents with more flexibility in their responses yet still provide a series of most likely response options. Additionally, it is important to note that open-ended survey items are often a poor choice for survey designers interested in collecting the kind of rich, descriptive data needed for credible qualitative research.[30] Therefore, if there are more than just a few open-ended response items, the survey designer should strongly reconsider whether a survey is the right study method (see **Step 1: Needs Assessment**).

In addition to the considerations discussed previously in this section, Table 7 provides recommendations for how to write high-quality items; it also provides solutions for several common pitfalls. Further, Appendix 2 provides a comprehensive checklist of item-writing guidelines to consider.

Visually Displaying Items

After items have been developed and response options selected, there are still several considerations regarding the visual presentation of the items with their respective response options. The platform used to administer the survey (e.g., computer, smartphone, paper, etc.) will often dictate an appropriate visual presentation. Web-based platforms allow for additional formats (e.g., drop down menus) that are not easily represented on paper-based surveys. In general, items should be arranged in either columns or rows (but not both), and columns may be preferable for web-based formats that may use smartphones for completion.[31,32] Fig. 3 illustrates some common visual design challenges to consider when formatting survey items.

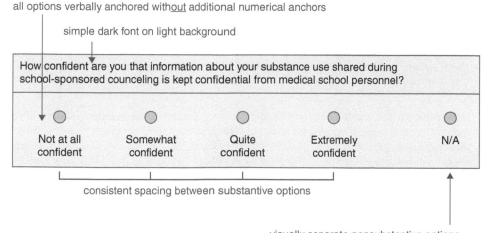

all options verbally anchored without additional numerical anchors

simple dark font on light background

How confident are you that information about your substance use shared during school-sponsored counceling is kept confidential from medical school personnel?

| Not at all confident | Somewhat confident | Quite confident | Extremely confident | N/A |

consistent spacing between substantive options

visually separate nonsubstantive options

Fig. 3 Visual Design Recommendations.

Testing Items

After a set of survey items has been drafted following the basic tenets of good item writing, there are some additional steps that may further clarify the items and improve respondents' cognitive response processes. Many of these advanced techniques begin to cross into survey validation; however, the discussion in this chapter focuses only on how these techniques can improve the quality of the items as applied to the cognitive response model. Two common approaches are expert reviews and cognitive interviewing; both should be performed.

EXPERT REVIEWS

Expert reviews are a pretesting technique that begins to address an important source of validity evidence: survey content. This technique involves selecting a variety of experts who closely review the draft survey and rate the items based on a set of criteria laid out by the survey designers (see Appendix 4). These criteria may include, for example, the clarity of the items, the relevance of the items to the construct being assessed, and identification of any missing items or concepts.[19] The clarity of the items is directly related to how well the experts believe respondents will comprehend the items, and expert reviews may uncover item language and/or syntax that could potentially confuse respondents. Relevance provides information about the extent to which experts believe a particular item is related to the survey construct. Finally, expert review forms often include an area for experts to provide input on additional items that may be considered relevant to the construct but have been omitted in the initial survey draft. The inclusion of items unrelated to the construct, or the exclusion of items that are related to the construct, can have negative impacts on the content validity of the survey.

Depending on the needs of the survey designer and the overarching purpose of the survey, it may be important to create rating scales for each of the criteria being assessed by the experts and then to set a predetermined cut point for what defines acceptability (see Appendix 4). This process allows the survey designer to systematically collect information about things like item clarity and relevance. Designers can use these rating scales to assess interrater agreement among experts and determine the extent to which their ratings are reliable. Doing so helps the survey designer determine what to do with each item (i.e., revise, remove, or replace). For more on how to quantify the expert review process, readers are encouraged to consult additional resources.[33-35]

VOICE OF EXPERIENCE

Although content experts know a lot about their areas of focus, they are typically not well trained in survey design. And although they may be quite good at identifying content problems (e.g., relevance of the items to the construct), they may be unskilled at identifying poorly written items or response scales that might induce biased answers. Thus, consulting both content and survey-design experts during the expert review process is often considered a best practice.

Experts can be content experts, survey-design experts, and/or analysis experts, and the selection of the experts often begins with local individuals at the survey designer's home institution who may have expertise in the area of interest. They should be third-party individuals who were not previously involved with the survey creation. Additionally, soliciting individuals with expertise external to the institution can be an effective way to improve the reviewer pool and ultimately the quality of survey items. A list of content experts can often be generated by reviewing the authorship lines in manuscripts reviewed during the literature search. Although there is no defined number of experts that must be used, having more than 10 can be useful if the survey designer hopes to conduct the review in a quantitative way, using rating scales and specific cut scores.[34] Alternatively, the expert review can be conducted in more of a qualitative way, with open-ended comments from just a handful of experts (i.e., fewer than 10).

COGNITIVE INTERVIEWS

Conducting cognitive interviews with individuals from the target population is another important step in collecting evidence related to response process validity. As was described earlier in the cognitive response process model, an important threat to the overall quality of a survey is whether respondents interpret items in the way the survey designer intended. The cognitive interview provides a way to test the degree to which respondents go through the response process model (comprehension, retrieval, judgment/estimation, response) with the intent of identifying potential sources of error in specific processes.[36]

VOICE OF EXPERIENCE

It is good practice to keep a running log of items that were added or removed from the survey, in addition to the rationale for these changes, throughout the expert review and cognitive interviewing processes. A running log provides valuable information about the development and evolution of the survey instrument over time, and it can be incredibly useful when it is time to draft the "Methods" and "Results" sections of the resulting manuscript.

Two different approaches, *think-aloud* and *verbal probing*, are the most common techniques. Moreover, the two techniques can be combined as an initial think-aloud followed by further probing of responses. That said, either approach alone can provide sufficient information to discover or confirm problematic items and improve the overall survey flow.

Think-Aloud Approach

The think-aloud approach encourages respondents to explicitly verbalize their thinking as they arrive at a particular answer choice, and this verbalization allows for a better understanding of how and the degree to which respondents move through all (or some) of the steps in the cognitive response process model. A potential disadvantage to using this approach exclusively is that respondents may not spontaneously verbalize their entire thought process. What is more, think-aloud protocols tend to generate excessive verbal data, and the task of analyzing that (often meandering) data can be quite overwhelming for many survey designers.

Verbal Probing Approach

A more focused approach to cognitive interviewing is to use verbal probing, whereby the interviewer obtains specific information from the respondent through a set of predetermined probing questions.[37] Some typical cognitive interview questions include, for example:

1. *What is the question trying to find out from you?*
2. *Can you repeat the question in your own words?*
3. *Which answer would you choose as the right answer for you?*
4. *How sure are you about your answer?*
5. *Can you explain to me how you came up with that answer?*
6. *I noticed that you hesitated. Tell me what you were thinking?*
7. *Tell me more about that...*

Again, this approach allows for specific information to be gathered about how respondents comprehend each item and where ambiguity may exist and about how information is retrieved and processed into a final judgment. Verbal probing can be done using either concurrent or retrospective probes. *Concurrent probing* entails the interviewer asking questions about the respondent's thought process as she or he responds to each item, which can be quite disruptive. That said, concurrent probes allow for immediate, in-the-moment responses that can also be quite informative. *Retrospective probing* moves the questions about a respondent's thought process to the end of the survey or a particular section of the survey and tends to be much less disruptive. However, with retrospective probing, there is an increased risk of recall bias and incomplete recollection of all thought processes.[38] Taken together, verbal probing is a powerful technique, although frequent interruptions on the part of the interviewer can have the effect of altering how a respondent would normally approach a particular item or section of the survey.

Performing Cognitive Interviews

With proper training, cognitive interviews can be conducted by anyone planning to administer a survey. All that is needed to conduct a cognitive interview is a quiet place, an audio recorder, and an interviewer script consisting of the verbal probes to be asked during the interview. When selecting subjects, survey designers should look for individuals who are similar to the target survey population. Useful cognitive interviewing data can be attained by selecting a few members of the target audience; the sample can be as few as five or six individuals or as many as several dozen, depending on time and resources.[19] Although there is typically no need to achieve any type of statistical representation when recruiting subjects, the goal is usually to pretest the survey using a diverse range of individuals within the practical constraints of time and cost.[37] The qualitative data from the cognitive interviews are then used to inform item and survey-wide revisions, with the ultimate goal of finding problems before the survey is launched, thus creating a set of high-quality items structured in a well-organized, understandable survey.

Survey Construction Checklist

☐ Consider the fundamental decision points for each item.
  ☐ Appropriate language for sampling frame
  ☐ Question vs. Statement stem
  ☐ Response option types
  ☐ Number of response options
  ☐ Nonsubstantive response options
  ☐ Item polarity
  ☐ Open-ended items
☐ Review each item for potential pitfalls in the cognitive response process model.
  ☐ Comprehension
  ☐ Retrieval
  ☐ Judgment/Estimation
  ☐ Response
☐ Send a draft instrument for expert review.
  ☐ Content experts
  ☐ Survey experts
  ☐ Other stakeholders
☐ Perform cognitive interviews.
  ☐ Think-aloud approach
  ☐ Verbal probing approach
☐ Conduct small pilot study.

References

1. Tourangeau R. The survey response process from a cognitive viewpoint. *Quality Assurance in Education.* 2018;26(2):169–181.
2. Jabine T, Straf ML, Tanur JM, Tourangeau R, eds. *Cognitive Aspects of Survey Design: Building a Bridge Between Discipline.* Washington, DC: National Academies Press; 1984: 73-100.
3. DeMaio T, Landreth A. Do different cognitive interview techniques produce different results? In: Presser S, Rothgeb JM, Couper MP, Lessler JT, Martin E, Martin J, Singer E, eds. *Methods for Testing and Evaluating Survey Questionnaire.* Hoboken, NJ: Wiley; 2004:891–908.
4. Tourangea R, Rips LJ, Rasinski K. *The Psychology of Survey Response.* Cambridge, UK: Cambridge University Press; 2000.
5. Schwarz N, Bless H. Constructing reality and its alternatives: assimilation and contrast effects in social judgment. In Hillsdale NJ, Martin LL, Tesser A, eds. *The Construction of Social Judgments.* 1992:217–245.
6. Burton S, Blair E. Task conditions, response formulation processes, and response accuracy for behavioral frequency questions in surveys. *Public Opin Q.* 1999;55(1):50–79.
7. Galesic M, Tourangeau R, Couper MP, Conrad FG. Eye-tracking data: new insights on response order effects and other cognitive shortcuts in survey responding. *Public Opin Q.* 2008;72(5):892–913.
8. Krosnick JA. Survey research. *Annu Rev Psychol.* 1999;50:537–567.
9. Krosnick JA. Response strategies for coping with the cognitive demands of attitude measures in surveys. *Appl Cognitive Psychol 1991.* 1991;5(3):213–236.
10. Tourangeau R, Sun H, Conrad FG, Couper MP. Examples in open-ended survey questions. *Int J Public Opin Res.* 2017;29(4):690–702.
11. Peytchev A, Conrad F, Couper M, Tourangeau R. Increasing respondents' use of definitions in web surveys. *J Official Stat.* 2010;26(4):633–650.
12. Leech GN. *Principles of Pragmatics.* New York: Pearson; 1983.
13. Costa PT, McCrae RR. From catalog to classification: Murray's needs and the five-factor model. *J Pers Soc Psychol.* 1988;55:258–265.
14. Goldberg LR. An alternative "description of personality": the big-five factor structure. *J Pers Soc Psychol.* 1990;9: 491-401.
15. Gehlbach H, Artino Jr AR. The Survey Checklist (Manifesto). *Acad Med. 2018*;93:360–366.
16. Saris WE, Revilla M, Krosnick JA, Shaeffer EM. Comparing questions with agree/disagree response option to questions with item-specific response options. *Surv Res Methods.* 2010;4:61–79.
17. Digman JM. Personality structure: emergence of the five-factor model. *Annu Rev Psychol.* 1990;41: 417–440.
18. Gehlbach H. Seven survey sins. *J Early Adolesc.* 2015;35:883–897.
19. Artino AR, LaRochelle JS, DeZee KJ, Gehlbach H. Developing questionnaires for educational research: AMEE Guide No. 87. *Med Teach.* 2014;36:463–474.
20. Elig TW, Frieze IH. Measuring causal attributions for success and failure. *J Pers Soc Psychol.* 1979;37(4):621–634.
21. Miethe TD. The validity and reliability of value measurements. *J Psychol.* 1985;119(5):441–453.
22. Groves RM, Dillman DA, Eltinge JL, Little RJA, eds. *Survey Nonresponse.* Hoboken, NJ: Wiley; 2002.
23. Dillman DA, Smyth JD, Christian LM. *Internet, Phone, Mail, and Mixed-Mode Surveys: The Tailored Design Method.* 4th ed. Hoboken, NJ: Wiley; 2014.
24. Cook DA, Beckman TJ. Does scale length matter? A comparison of nine- versus five-point rating scales for the mini-CEX. *Adv Heal Sci Educ Theory Pract.* 2009;14:655–664.
25. Weng L-J. Impact of the number of response categories and anchor labels on coefficient alpha and test-retest reliability. *Educ Psychol Meas.* 2004;64:956–972.
26. Christian LM, Dillman DA. The influence of graphical and symbolic language manipulations on responses to self-administered questions. *Public Opin Q.* 2004;68(1):57–80.
27. Stern MJ, Dillman DA, Smyth JD. Visual design, order effects, and respondent characteristics in a self-administered survey. *Surv Res Methods.* 2007;1(3):1–11.
28. Israel GD. Effects of answer space size on responses to open-ended questions in mail surveys. *J Official Stat.* 2010;26(2):271.
29. Chaudhary AK, Israel GD. Influence of importance statements and box size on response rate and response quality of open-ended questions in web/mail mixed-mode surveys. *J Rural Soc Sci.* 2016;31(3):140–159.

30. LaDonna KA, Taylor T, Lingard L. Why open-ended survey questions are unlikely to support rigorous qualitative insights. *Acad Med.* 2018;93(3):347–349.
31. De Bruijne M, Wijnant A. Improving response rates and questionnaire design for mobile web surveys. *Public Opin Q.* 2014;78:951–962.
32. Christian LM, Parsons NL, Dillman DA. Designing scalar questions for Web surveys. *Sociol Methods Res.* 2014;37:393–425.
33. Mccoach DB, Gable RK, Madura JP. *Instrument Development in the Affective Domain: School and Corporate Applications.* 3rd ed. New York: Springer; 2013.
34. Rubio DM, Berg-Weger M, Tebb SS, Lee ES, Ruach S. Objectifying content validity: conducting a content validity study in social work research. *Soc Work Res.* 2003;27(2):94–104.
35. McKenzie JF, Wood ML, Kotecki JE, Clark JK, Brey RA. Research notes. *Am J Health Behav.* 1999;23(4):311–318.
36. Karabenick SA, Woolley ME, Friedel JM, Ammon BV, Blazevski J, Bonney CR, De Groot E, Gilbert MC, Musu I, Kempler TM, Kelly KI. Cognitive processing of self-report items in educational research: do they think what we mean? *Educ Psychol.* 2007;42(3):139–151.
37. Willis GB, Artino AR. What do our respondents think we're asking? Using cognitive interviewing to improve medical education surveys. *J Grad Med Educ.* 2013;5(3):353–356.
38. Drennen J. Cognitive interviewing: verbal data in the design and pretesting of questionnaires. *J Adv Nurs.* 2003;42(1):57–63.

Establishing Evidence

David A. Cook, MD, MHPE

CHAPTER OUTLINE

At some point in survey development, the question will (or at least should) arise: Do the results have sufficient validity evidence? The topic of validity often strikes fear into the hearts of survey designers (researchers and educators). Although validity cannot be ignored, it need not be complicated or distressing. This chapter will demystify validity and describe a practical approach to collect evidence to support the validity of survey findings. It is a bit different from other chapters in this book because an explanation of conceptual underpinnings is needed before we get to the practical steps. The conceptual review is still quite brief; other sources offer a more comprehensive discussion.[1–5] This chapter first describes the concepts that support the three main validity frameworks, then goes into some detail on how to approach reliability, and concludes with a step-by-step approach to validation that is illustrated with the example survey (see **Book Introduction**) used throughout the book.

Validity, Validation, and Evidence

Validity is formally defined as "the degree to which evidence and theory support the interpretations of [scores] entailed by proposed uses,"[4] but for practical purposes it is best viewed in terms of the defensibility of the survey findings. If survey designers were called upon to defend the results in a court of law or to a group of friends, what could they say to convince the listeners that the results are credible? They might describe the careful process of generating, pilot testing, and revising items; note that the answers to items on a given topic generally clustered in a way that made sense (i.e., a pattern of consistently high or low responses from a given individual); or report that a small validation study prior to the formal survey found that respondents answered questions similarly when resurveyed after a 1-week delay, and that two subscales showed strong correlation with scores from another (longer) instrument that was not part of the final survey. The survey designer might also point out that the results are probably relevant only to the specific sample of respondents (e.g., physicians in Australia), and admit that it would have been better if the instrument had included some questions about a specific issue of national policy.

This brief example illustrates a few important points. First, validity is not a property of an instrument; the same instrument might provide valid (useful, credible) results when administered to practicing physicians in Australia, but yield erroneous or simply nonsensical results if administered to nurse practitioners, medical students, or physicians in another country. Thus it is not appropriate to talk about "valid instruments" (even though people, including well-known scholars, often do this); rather, we should talk about valid scores (or results) or more specifically about *valid inferences, conclusions, or decisions* that are made based on the scores and typically applied in a specific context.

Second, validity is not an all-or-nothing verdict. Scores might be sufficiently valid to support some conclusions but not others; for example, a political survey might correctly reflect the opinions of one political party but not the opinions of the entire population. Some jurors (or friends) might be convinced, whereas others remain doubtful.

Third, the procedures and empiric findings described earlier constitute *evidence* that supports the validity of the survey results. In trying to convince people, it helps to organize the evidence and present a coherent, honest, and complete summary. We call this the *validity argument*.

Finally, when articulating the argument, it is helpful to present multiple pieces of validity evidence.

So, validity is an evidence-based argument, and *validation* refers to the process of planning, collecting, and interpreting that evidence. We often read or speak of "validated instruments," but the label "validated" only tells us that a validation process has been applied. It does not tell us anything about which process was used, let alone the results (perhaps the evidence was unfavorable), the context/population, or the decisions that were validated.

 VOICE OF EXPERIENCE

Never talk about "valid instruments" or "validated instruments." More accurate wording might be: "The instrument scores justify valid interpretations [or conclusions or decisions] in this context," or "Evidence supports the validity of score interpretations for the purpose of...," or simply, "Score validity is supported by evidence showing..."

Validity Evidence and Validation Frameworks

Evidence to support the validity argument can come from various sources. Crafting a persuasive validity argument requires thoughtful planning. Several frameworks exist to guide the development of such plans. Discussed in this section are the classical framework, the five sources (Messick's) framework, and the four inferences (Kane's) framework.

TABLE 8 ■ The Classical Validity Framework

Type of Validity	Definition	Examples of Evidence
Content	Survey items constitute a relevant and representative sample of the domain being measured.	Procedures for item development and sampling
Criterion (includes correlational, concurrent, and predictive validity)	Correlation between the survey responses and some (usually hypothetical) "truth" (criterion).	Correlation with a definitive standard
Construct	Responses vary as expected based on an underlying psychological construct (used when no definitive criterion exists).	Correlation with another measure of the same construct Factor analysis Change or stability (depending on the situation) over time or across subgroups

CLASSICAL FRAMEWORK

The "classical" validation framework identified at least three different "types" of validity: *content*, *construct*, and *criterion* (with criterion having several subdivisions); see Table 8. *Reliability* is also part of this framework, although it is typically not viewed as a type of validity. Some people include *"face validity"* as a fourth type of validity. However, face validity is really not a separate form of validity.[2,6] Some concepts that are labeled face validity are really content validity; the rest are typically superficial appearances that have no bearing on the defensibility of the survey findings.

VOICE OF EXPERIENCE

Don't talk about "face validity." It's either "content validity" (or better: "content evidence") or irrelevant.

The classical framework, although familiar to many, is problematic and limited. First, at the end of the day there is really only one "type" of validity: the validity of the inference being made. The concepts of content, construct, and criterion validity are best viewed as different sources of evidence that support the overall validity. Second, *reliability* is generally agreed to be crucial in instrument validation, yet it does not neatly belong with any of the three validity types. Third, experts have identified additional sources of validity evidence not reflected in these concepts, such that this framework is incomplete. This framework remains commonly used, and it isn't wrong to use it; but the other, more contemporary frameworks described in the next sections are generally preferred.

FIVE SOURCES (MESSICK'S) FRAMEWORK

What is now commonly known as the "five sources" framework was first proposed by Messick in 1989 and subsequently adopted (after some modifications) as a standard for the field by the American Educational Research Association (AERA), the American Psychological Association, and the National Council on Measurement in Education in 1999 (and reaffirmed in 2014).[4] This framework identifies five sources of validity evidence[2,4,7] that correspond in part with the classical framework (see Table 9).

TABLE 9 ■ **The Five Sources of Evidence Validity Framework**

Source of Evidence	Definition	Examples of Evidence
Content	"The relationship between the content of a test and the construct it is intended to measure."[4]	Procedures for developing items, response options, and scoring rubric (e.g., expert panel, previously described instrument, test blueprint, pilot testing)
Internal structure	Relationship among items within the survey and how these relate to what is being measured.	Internal consistency reliability Interrater reliability Factor analysis
Relationships with other variables	"Degree to which these relationships are consistent with the construct underlying the proposed test score interpretations."[4]	Correlation with another measure of the same construct Change or stability (depending on the situation) over time or across subgroups
Response process	"The fit between the construct and the detailed nature of performance... actually engaged in."[4]	Analysis of respondents' thoughts or actions during assessment (e.g., think-aloud protocol) Survey quality control, security
Consequences	"The impact, beneficial or harmful and intended or unintended, of assessment."[16]	Impact of assessment on learning, direct (e.g., test-enhanced learning) or indirect (encouragement to study, support of tailored feedback) Success of remediation guided by assessment results Impact on teachers (e.g., motivation to improve teaching skills or revise course objectives)

See the next section for further details and examples.[2,7,17]

The first three sources of evidence are analogous to concepts found in the classical framework. *Content evidence* is essentially the same as the old concept of content validity. It consists of procedures that optimize the likelihood that survey items (including both questions and response options) clearly and completely capture the domains or concepts of interest (which we call *constructs*). *Internal structure evidence* uses reliability analysis, factor analysis, and analysis of score distributions (item analysis and differential item functioning) to evaluate the relationships of individual assessment items with each other and with the intended construct(s). *Relationships with other variables evidence* evaluates the associations between survey results and other measures or respondent demographics. These analyses correspond closely with classical notions of criterion validity and construct validity.

The other two sources of evidence in the "five sources" framework introduce concepts not found in the classical framework. First, *response process evidence* evaluates how respondents actually comprehend and answer questions (i.e., their thought processes), to uncover potential mismatches with the survey intent. Issues that might interfere with the quality of responses include poorly worded instructions or questions, confusing or misleading formatting, and the framing (range and wording) of response options (see **Step 2: Survey Construction**). Finally, *consequences evidence* looks at the impact (beneficial or harmful) of the survey on the target audience. As viewed through the lens of consequences, one indication of the ultimate validity of

TABLE 10 ■ **The Four Inferences Validity Framework**

Validity Inference	Definition (Assumptions)*	Examples of Evidence
Scoring	The score or written narrative from a given observation adequately captures key aspects of performance.	Procedures for creating and empirically evaluating item wording, response options, and scoring options Rater selection and training
Generalization	The total score or synthesis of narratives reflects performance across the test domain.	Sampling strategy (e.g., test blueprint) and sample size Internal consistency reliability Interrater reliability
Extrapolation	The total score or synthesis of narrative data obtained in the test setting reflects meaningful performance in a real-life setting.	Authenticity of context Correlation with tests measuring similar constructs, especially in real-life context Correlation (or lack thereof) with tests measuring different constructs Expert-novice comparisons Factor analysis (conceptual alignment with the proposed construct)
Implications/Decisions	Measured performance constitutes a rational basis for meaningful decisions and actions.	See Table 9, "Consequences."

Note: See Kane[5] and Cook et al.[3] for further details and examples.
*Each of the inferences reflects an assumption about the creation and use of assessment results.

survey results is the degree to which the findings lead to meaningful, desired change. Although the five sources framework is comprehensive in identifying possible sources of evidence, it provides little guidance on how to prioritize the evidence that might be most important in a given situation.

FOUR INFERENCES (KANE'S) FRAMEWORK

The third and most recently developed validity framework, Kane's "four inferences" framework (Table 10), helps survey designers logically organize and prioritize the evidence needed. However, to accomplish this, it avoids completely the concepts and terminology of the classical and five sources frameworks and introduces an entirely new paradigm. Thus, when first learning the four inferences framework, it helps to simply disregard the older frameworks and start with a clean slate rather than attempt to map the older frameworks onto Kane's.

 VOICE OF EXPERIENCE

When learning the four inferences framework, it is best to start with a clean slate rather than try to map the classical or five sources concepts onto the four inferences. It simply does not work neatly.

In essence, the four inferences represent key stages during the survey process in which error (invalidity) can be introduced, starting with the observation of whatever is being measured, and ending with the consequences or impact of the survey results. A survey item is designed to measure something: a belief, a past or anticipated event (e.g., prescribing a medication), a characteristic (e.g., height) or aptitude (e.g., knowledge), etc. Let's call a single opportunity to measure this something an *observation*. The respondent makes a response (e.g., Likert-type, multiple-choice, free-text narrative) that we assume is an accurate measure of this observation. Responses to several items are often combined to generate what we assume is a more complete picture of whatever is being observed (from the respondent's perspective); this in turn is assumed to reflect some semblance of reality; and then this representation of reality is assumed to constitute a rational basis for making a decision and taking action. For example, in measuring anxiety, a single self-report item is scored; this item's score is combined with other item scores to form a total score that we presume reflects the clinical state of anxiety, and this score is used to make a decision about referral for psychiatric support.

Of course, there are many reasons why these assumptions probably are never entirely true; thus each of these four steps represents an inference that might be incorrect. The respondent's documentation of the observation (the *scoring inference*) could be flawed because of an inaccurate perception or a faulty documentation procedure; the combination of several responses (the *generalization inference*) could be flawed if the responses collectively omit an important aspect of the observation; even if accurate for these observations, this combination of responses could be flawed contextually if it is not a complete and accurate representation of the entire scope of relevant reality (*extrapolation inference*); and even this could be flawed if it does not provide information relevant to making the decision at hand (*implications/decision* inference). Kane's framework evaluates each of these four inferences in turn and suggests evidence that can be used to test how well the corresponding assumptions hold up. This approach guides survey designers to prioritize the weakest links in the chain of inferences, which is better than starting with evidence sources and working backward. Note that this prioritization does not necessarily follow the sequence of inferences (e.g., evidence to support scoring does not necessarily receive higher priority than evidence to support generalization). Those who want to learn more about the four inferences framework should refer to additional sources.[3,8]

SELECTING AMONG THE FRAMEWORKS

None of these frameworks is inherently "best" or currently viewed as a universal standard, so how is a framework chosen? Although the AERA established the five sources framework as the standard for the field, all three are currently used; and this remains an individual choice that balances the strengths and weaknesses of each approach. The classical framework suffers from both conceptual and practical limitations but has the benefit of widespread use and shared understanding. The five sources framework resolves many of these limitations and retains several concepts of the classical framework, which facilitates communication with audiences familiar only with the classical framework; but the five sources still lack a clear approach to prioritize evidence. The four inferences framework has the advantage of helping survey designers prioritize the evidence needed; but this framework represents an entirely new paradigm and introduces concepts that do not directly correspond to those in the other two frameworks, which can impair adoption.

 VOICE OF EXPERIENCE

When choosing among frameworks, consider your audience (With which framework will they be most familiar? What types of evidence will they expect and understand?), the complexity and completeness required of the final validity argument (more robust validation efforts will require a more contemporary framework), and your own skill and comfort. If possible, it is recommended to use one of the more contemporary frameworks (five sources or four inferences).

Internal Structure and Generalization

The evidence to support internal structure (in the five sources framework) and generalization (in the four inferences framework) most often comes from analyses evaluating the reliability and factor structure of scores. *Reliability* and *factor analysis* are also important in the classical framework, but (as noted earlier) don't fit neatly with any of the three validity types.

RELIABILITY

Reliability is generally considered an essential element of robust assessment—a necessary but not independently sufficient source of validity evidence. Reliability refers to the reproducibility or consistency of scores across two or more observations that purport to measure the same construct. The word "*observation*" can refer to a variety of assessment events, including the response to a single survey or test item (e.g., multiple-choice question); performance on one skill station; ratings from one skill station supervisor; or total scores from one test. When we look at the reliability (reproducibility) across several of these events, we attach labels such as internal consistency (across items), interstation reliability (across stations), inter-rater reliability (across raters), and test-retest reliability (across the same test administered on a subsequent date). A given observation often consists of several conditions that are or could be replicated (e.g., a clinical skills exam might consist of several stations, each with several raters, each using a rating form with several items); we call these conditions (stations, raters, items) *facets* of the observation.

 VOICE OF EXPERIENCE

Although people often speak of "validity and reliability," it is important to recognize that reliability is just one of several sources of validity evidence and is ideally considered part of a comprehensive validity argument framed using the five sources or four inferences framework.

When thinking about how to analyze reliability, it is helpful to ask two questions: 1) What is changing from one observation to the next? and 2) Are these observations purporting to measure the same construct? Regarding question 1, it is essential to be clear about what facet(s) is (are) changing: the items, stations, raters, dates, or something else. Multiple facets can be present simultaneously. For example, a five-item checklist used by two raters at each of three stations in a skills exam could generate measures of inter-item reliability (known as "internal consistency"), inter-rater reliability, and inter-station reliability. Simply talking about "reliability" in this situation would leave readers confused. Moreover, focusing on only one of these reliabilities would be insufficient in most situations.

The second question (whether observations measure the same construct) is even more important, and often more difficult to answer. For some assessments, such as a multiple-choice test of knowledge or a questionnaire to measure well-being, the construct being measured is obvious, and the answer to question 2 is straightforward. In other situations, and commonly in survey research, the answer is less obvious. For example, question 12 in a hypothetical survey might ask, "How often do you use online learning?" and question 13 might ask, "How often do you use simulation task trainers for learning?" Are the constructs addressed in these items–online learning and simulation task trainers– the same (i.e., both are types of "educational technologies")? Or are they different (i.e., use of online learning is really quite different from use of task trainers)? The answer depends on the overall purpose of the survey and the message the survey designer is trying to communicate. If viewed as different, then calculating inter-item reliability for these items does not make sense.

VOICE OF EXPERIENCE

Survey designers often define an instrument as reflecting multiple subscales or domains, each measuring a distinct construct (sometimes even supporting this with empiric evidence, e.g., factor analysis) and then go on to report the inter-item reliability for scores from all instrument items together. This usually doesn't make sense and should generally be avoided. As a guiding principle, reliability should be reported for each subscale individually, rather than for all items in the instrument. An exception is when the subscales collectively address a broader but still recognizable construct (e.g., a test of "cardiology knowledge" could have subscales of ischemic heart disease, electrophysiology, and heart failure; and it would be reasonable to report reliability for the test as a whole and for each subscale).

Although reliability is important, remember that it contributes only one form of evidence (internal structure [in the five sources framework] or generalization [in the four inferences framework]), and in survey research this might not even be among the most important sources of evidence. Also, reliability—like validity—is a property of scores (not instruments).

Reliability is usually reported as a reliability coefficient[9] ranging from 0 to 1. The reliability coefficient can be interpreted as the correlation between scores from at least two observations (two items, raters, stations, etc.). There are several ways to calculate the reliability coefficient, but the most important distinction among the various approaches is how many observations are presumed to be included in the final score. For example, for a 20-item multiple-choice question exam, we usually take the average across all questions to calculate the final score for that exam and so calculate the reliability across all 20 items; but we could also consider each item individually. Alternatively, if two raters score 20% of a series of videotaped procedural tasks and a single rater scores the remaining 80%, it would usually be useful to know the reliability for the single rater; yet sometimes it might be interesting to know the reliability if instead we used the average score of both raters. Some reliability coefficients (such as Cronbach alpha) indicate the reliability of many observations (e.g., all the items on the exam), whereas others (such as kappa) indicate the reliability estimated for a single observation (e.g., single rater). There are also methods such as the Spearman-Brown formula that allow conversion from one number of observations to another (e.g., calculating the reliability for four raters instead of two). When reporting a reliability coefficient, it is essential to specify the number of observations included.

These conventions are not universal; it would be perfectly acceptable (and in some situations, desirable) to report the single-item reliability in a multiple-choice exam or inter-rater reliability for a group of raters. However, these choices have implications for our interpretation of the reliability coefficient because reliability (nearly always) improves with more observations. For Cronbach's alpha, a value of >0.7 is commonly accepted as a minimum acceptable value, and >0.8 is generally desirable.[10] By contrast, for kappa a value >0.2 is considered "fair," >0.4 is "moderate," and >0.6 is "substantial."[11] Do not confuse these interpretation thresholds! Moreover, these thresholds should not be confused with those used for interpreting traditional correlation coefficients (e.g., Pearson's r), for which a value >0.3 is classified as "medium" and >0.5 is classified as "large."[12] Finally, note that a very high reliability (e.g., Cronbach's alpha >0.9) could suggest an opportunity to reduce the number of items (perhaps using principal components analysis as suggested later in the next section).

FACTOR STRUCTURE

Factor analysis[13] is used to investigate relationships between the items in an instrument and the intended constructs. Factor analysis can empirically determine the extent to which items that are intended to measure a given construct actually cluster together. Confirmation of expected clustering supports (but does not prove) that the items are measuring a similar construct (which we presume to be the intended construct). In contrast, failure to confirm expected clustering (e.g., if items "load" on the wrong cluster ["factor"] or cross-load on several factors) suggests that the items might not be measuring the intended construct. Although factor analysis is an essential part of many validation plans, it may or may not be relevant to a survey instrument for the same reason that inter-item reliability may or may not be relevant. A survey that measures one or several defined constructs (e.g., burnout, attitudes about patient safety, or knowledge of quality improvement methodologies) might warrant factor analysis. Conversely, factor analysis probably doesn't make sense for a survey composed of multiple conceptually distinct items (e.g., frequency of use of 15 different electronic knowledge resources, or ratings of user-friendliness of 12 different social media apps).

Principal components analysis is another method used to investigate relationships between the items in an instrument and the intended constructs, conceptually similar to (and often confused with) factor analysis but serving a distinct purpose. Whereas factor analysis evaluates item clustering (the underlying factor structure), principal components analysis is used to determine whether the instrument can be shortened by removing less relevant items without a substantial sacrifice in measurement quality. As with factor analysis, principal components analysis may or may not be relevant to a given survey instrument. Readers can refer to other sources for further details on factor analysis and principal components analysis.[13-15]

Crafting the Arguments: Planning, Prioritizing, and Interpreting the Evidence

As noted earlier, validity is best viewed as an evidence-based argument. There are two distinct stages of this argument: the up-front planning of what evidence to collect, and then the appraisal or synthesis of actual evidence into a concise summary and bottom line. Kane calls the up-front planning the "interpretation-use argument" (IUA), and the final appraisal the "validity argument."

Planning and appraising these arguments require us to prioritize the evidence that is most needed, and this requires us to identify the weakest links (most tenuous assumptions). It is not just the quantity of evidence that matters, but also the relevance, quality, and breadth. For example (using the four inferences framework): Which aspects of scoring are most questionable (e.g., respondents' memories, the choice of response options, survey security—such as for cheating)? Which aspects of generalization (e.g., item sampling and wording, reliability, domain factor structure), extrapolation (e.g., item sampling, representation of real-world problems), and implications (e.g., relevance to decision making) are most critical? It is helpful at this stage to identify as many assumptions as possible and then to prioritize these. The same task can be approached from the perspective of the five evidence sources framework, too: Which aspects of content, response process, internal structure, etc. would be most useful in constructing a coherent argument? Regardless of approach, the final prioritized list of assumptions and desired evidence constitutes the IUA. Specifying the IUA is analogous to stating a research hypothesis and articulating the evidence required to empirically test that hypothesis.

Once evidence has been collected as outlined in the IUA, the survey designer organizes and synthesizes this evidence into a validity argument, a succinct summary of the empiric findings, and how they agree or disagree with projections. It is usually appropriate for the survey designer to make an overall judgment of validity for the intended use (e.g., strongly supported, weakly supported, inconclusive, or undermined), but sufficient detail should always be reported as to allow readers to form their own judgment.

Using, Modifying, and Combining Existing Instruments

It is extremely common and appropriate—even advisable—to incorporate all or part of an existing instrument when creating a new survey. Evidence collected in a previous study for a given instrument's scores (by the same study leaders or by others) is always admissible into the validity argument, but its weight depends on at least two points. First, how similar were the previous study participants, context, and conditions to those of the present survey? Second, how similar is the intended use or decision in the previous and present study? Abundant favorable evidence across multiple contexts (multiple studies) will carry substantial weight, but existing evidence is (almost) never entirely sufficient. Survey designers should plan to strategically collect new evidence to fill gaps as guided by the IUA.

It is also very common to modify the item wording or response options, use only a subset of items, or combine part or all of several instruments into a single instrument. These and other modifications (such as modified instructions or different delivery modalities) can potentially have a significant impact (both practically and statistically significant!) on validity. Again, previous evidence is always admissible, but the relevance and weight will vary depending on the type and magnitude of modifications. It helps to consider in turn each source of validity evidence and the plausible impact of the modifications. For example, a change in instructions might change the response processes, whereas a change in the number of items would very likely alter the reliability. In some instances (e.g., with extensive changes to wording, use of a small subset of items, or mixing items from several instruments together), it is more appropriate to consider the instrument as entirely new. Fortunately, the initial grounding in an existing instrument or instruments stills counts as evidence (e.g., content evidence in the five-sources framework).

An Eight-Step Approach to Validation

Although the previously discussed concepts are essential to understanding the process of validation, it is also important to be able to apply this process in practical ways. Cook and Hatala outlined an eight-step approach to validation[1] that works with any of the validity frameworks described previously. This approach is outlined in the next section and illustrated by working through the example survey (see **Book Introduction** for the case) using the perspective of the five sources framework. This approach is rarely linear; rather, a robust validation will typically involve several cycles through some or all steps.

1. DEFINE THE CONSTRUCT(S) AND PROPOSED INTERPRETATION(S)

Validation begins by clarifying what is being measured. In our example, we need to clarify which aspect(s) of substance abuse we want to focus on: Are we measuring beliefs about substance abuse, personal history of substance abuse, knowledge of the effects of substance abuse, ability to counsel and frequency of counseling patients about substance abuse, or some combination of those aspects? Each of these aspects of the larger topic would require a rather different series of survey questions. Sometimes it is helpful to consider (and validate) each aspect separately, at least initially. However, at some point the instrument must be validated as a whole because the disparate sections can influence one another (e.g., asking questions about personal history early in the survey might influence responses to subsequent questions about beliefs). For the present example, we will assess the personal history of substance abuse.

2. MAKE EXPLICIT THE INTENDED DECISION(S)

Although it is crucial to clarify the proposed interpretation, perhaps the more relevant question is: What are we going to do with this information? Knowing this answer—the intended decision— will guide most of the other validation choices. Will we use this information to try to change government policies about substance abuse, uncover gaps in the school curriculum, or identify unmet needs for social support? For the example, we will focus on identifying unmet social support needs.

3. DEFINE THE INTERPRETATION-USE ARGUMENT AND PRIORITIZE NEEDED VALIDITY EVIDENCE

Interpreting scores and then making decisions entail multiple assumptions about what the numbers actually mean. We need to recognize these assumptions, prioritize them, and plan how to test them (i.e., What evidence can we collect to support or refute these assumptions?). This line of reasoning constitutes the IUA.[8]

For most surveys, robust content evidence is essential: How were the relevant domains (topics, themes, concepts, constructs), subdomains, and individual items selected? Who verified the wording of each item and the corresponding instructions? Why was one response option format selected over other possibilities? How extensive was the pilot testing, and how carefully was the instrument refined after pilot testing? All of these questions must be addressed.

Further planning of the IUA may require a clearer articulation of the survey purpose and component parts. For example, in considering the internal structure evidence: If the survey has items examining knowledge of substance abuse, it makes sense to calculate inter-item reliability for these items. Likewise, if the survey has items inquiring about attitudes regarding substance abuse, then both reliability and perhaps factor analysis might be useful. In contrast, items regarding the frequency of personal experience with various substances of abuse would probably not warrant either reliability or factor analysis. However, it may be possible to explore relationships with other variables by evaluating specific (hypothesized) relationships among knowledge, attitudes, personal experience, and other variables (e.g., year of training, family background). The result of this planning stage is a detailed map of the survey components, their predicted interrelationships, and (most important) what these relationships say about the validity of the decision; all of this can occur before survey items have even been created (let alone tested or used). Such planning often benefits from involvement of a statistician, psychometrician, or other experienced methodologist.

4. IDENTIFY CANDIDATE INSTRUMENTS AND/OR CREATE/ADAPT A NEW INSTRUMENT

Whenever possible, it helps to build from an existing instrument rather than start *de novo*. Sometimes a survey can simply adopt a previously used instrument intact; other times, several instruments (or selected items from one or more instruments) will be combined. To the extent that the original instrument was itself well developed, using all or part of it provides evidence of content. The very fact that other instruments were sought, the diligence of the search, and the process of screening and selecting candidate instruments also provide content evidence (i.e., evidence that the most appropriate instrument was identified, rather than simply selecting one with which the authors were already familiar). Selection might consider the relevance of the items, the context of prior use, and the nature of existing validity evidence. Even instruments that are not ultimately used can contribute to the development of new items by suggesting processes for item development, concepts and themes that might be measured, and specific approaches to item construction.

Although some items, response options, or instructions may require modification, all changes should be thoughtfully considered and minimized as much as possible. Strictly speaking, any modification (selecting, combining, reordering, or rewording items or instructions) creates a new instrument, and all previous evidence is (strictly speaking) irrelevant. In practice, it is nonetheless extremely useful (indeed, essential) to consider previous evidence; and the fewer the modifications, the smaller the logical leap in applying the evidence. See **Step 2: Survey Construction** for further details on instrument creation.

5. APPRAISE EXISTING EVIDENCE AND COLLECT NEW EVIDENCE AS NEEDED

If one or more previously used instruments is adopted, the validity evidence for each of these should be carefully identified and appraised: How well does available evidence fulfill the priorities identified in the IUA (validation step #3)? Modifying or combining instruments will naturally influence the relevance of this evidence, as will the specific context of the new survey. However, thoughtfully considering existing evidence will identify gaps and will often suggest approaches that will fill those gaps.

To the extent that the final instrument is new or modified or whether gaps exist in the current evidence base, new validity evidence will need to be collected, as guided by the IUA. This new evidence will typically come from a combination of pilot testing and data obtained during actual implementations.

Using our running example from the **Book Introduction**, if we are able to identify existing instruments with robust evidence of content and reliability, we can probably rely on the content evidence already existing for these instruments; moreover, a description of the sources searched in our process of discovering these instruments and the corresponding evidence can itself be entered as evidence. However, we will probably want to repeat the reliability and factor analyses as planned in validation step #3 and proceed with the newly proposed explorations of relationships with other variables.

6. KEEP TRACK OF PRACTICAL ISSUES INCLUDING COST

Although not directly relevant to the interpretation of scores, information about the practical issues surrounding development, implementation, and interpretation of scores will be important to survey designers (the original survey team and others who might wish to adopt the instrument for future use). The expense, technical expertise, and logistical challenges inherent in implementing the instrument will need to be considered against the usefulness of the information gained. In our example, we will want to track the cost of printing the survey for paper mail distribution and the charges for electronic survey preparation and administration.

7. FORMULATE/SYNTHESIZE THE VALIDITY ARGUMENT IN RELATION TO THE INTERPRETATION-USE ARGUMENT

After collecting validity evidence (validation step #5), this evidence should be synthesized and then contrasted with the evidence that was planned as part of the IUA. This final synthesis constitutes the validity argument.

8. MAKE A JUDGMENT: DOES EVIDENCE SUPPORT THE INTENDED USE?

The concluding step is to interpret the validity argument and render judgment regarding the degree to which intended interpretations and decisions are supported by the instrument scores.

Using our example, validation steps #7 and #8 will culminate in a final judgment of whether the scores reflect the knowledge, attitudes, and personal experiences of medical students regarding substance abuse sufficiently well that we can trust the results; and if not, then which element(s) of the survey should be interpreted with caution?

Reporting Validation Efforts

Survey designers often wonder how and where to report their validation results. There is no standard procedure, and indeed the answer may vary according to author and journal preferences. In general, content evidence (including a description of previously reported instruments and any previously reported validity evidence and of the development and final description of any newly developed items) is reported in the "Methods" section for most survey studies. Exceptions exist, of course: For studies that focus heavily on the instrument itself (i.e., validation studies) in addition to or instead of the survey findings, the description of prior instruments might be located in the "Introduction" (as background to justify the needs for the current validation effort); whereas if the study employed a robust quantitative approach to develop items, then these findings might be reported in the "Results" section.

For other sources of validity evidence, a helpful general principle is: If the validation was background to the main purpose of the study (e.g., the main purpose is to showcase the survey results), then most validation results probably fit best in the "Methods" section. In contrast, if validation is the main purpose of the study (e.g., developing and testing a new instrument), then validation results might best be reported in the "Results."

An Eight-Step Approach to Validation Summary

- ☐ Define the construct and proposed interpretation.
- ☐ Make explicit the intended decision(s).
- ☐ Define the IUA and prioritize needed validity evidence.
- ☐ Identify candidate instruments and/or create/adapt a new instrument.
- ☐ Appraise existing evidence and collect new evidence as needed.
- ☐ Keep track of practical issues, including cost.
- ☐ Formulate/synthesize the validity argument in relation to the IUA.
- ☐ Make a judgment: Does evidence support the intended use?

References

1. Cook DA, Hatala R. Validation of educational assessments: a primer for simulation and beyond. *Adv Simul (Lond)*. 2016;1:31.
2. Cook DA, Beckman TJ. Current concepts in validity and reliability for psychometric instruments: theory and application. *Am J Med*. 2006;119:166.e7-16.
3. Cook DA, Brydges R, Ginsburg S, Hatala R. A contemporary approach to validity arguments: a practical guide to Kane's framework. *Med Educ*. 2015;49:560–575.
4. American Educational Research Association, American Psychological Association, National Council on Measurement in Education. *Standards for Educational and Psychological Testing*. Washington, DC: American Educational Research Association; 2014: 11-31.
5. Kane MT. Validation. In: Brennan RL, ed. *Educational Measurement*. Westport, CT: Praeger; 2006: 17–64.
6. Downing SM. Face validity of assessments: faith-based interpretations or evidence-based science? *Med Educ*. 2006;40:7–8.
7. Cook DA, Zendejas B, Hamstra SJ, Hatala R, Brydges R. What counts as validity evidence? Examples and prevalence in a systematic review of simulation-based assessment. *Adv Health Sci Educ*. 2014;19:233–250.
8. Kane MT. Validating the *Interpretations and uses of test scores. J Educ Meas*. 2013;50:1–73.
9. Traub RE, Rowley GL. An NCME instructional module on understanding reliability. *Educational Measurement: Issues and Practice*. 1991;10(1):37–45.
10. Downing SM. Reliability: on the reproducibility of assessment data. *Med Educ*. 2004;38:1006–1012.
11. Landis J, Koch G. The measurement of observer agreement for categorical data. *Biometrics*. 1977;33: 159–174.
12. Cohen J. *Statistical Power Analysis for the Behavioral Sciences*. 2nd ed. Hillsdale, NJ: Lawrence Erlbaum; 1988.
13. Floyd FJ, Widaman KF. Factor analysis in the development and refinement of clinical assessment instruments. *Psychol Assess*. 1995;7:286–299.
14. Kline P. *An Easy Guide to Factor Analysis*. New York: Routledge; 1994.
15. Gorsuch RL. *Factor Analysis*. 2nd ed. Hillsdale, NJ: Lawrence Erlbaum; 1983.
16. Cook DA, Lineberry M. Consequences validity evidence: evaluating the impact of educational assessments. *Acad Med*. 2016;91:785–795.
17. Downing SM. Validity: on the meaningful interpretation of assessment data. *Med Educ*. 2003;37: 830–837.

STEP 4

Survey Delivery

Andrew W. Phillips, MD, MEd ▪ Steven J. Durning, MD, PhD ▪
Anthony R. Artino, Jr., PhD

There are many ways to administer a survey, from in-person interviews on the street corner to specialty apps downloaded by anyone in the world. The process that takes place from initial sending to receiving back a survey is fraught with opportunities to lose potential responses; this chapter walks through key points in the administration process and includes tips to maximize returns and minimize the burden on the survey designers (educators and researchers) and respondents. The first part of the delivery strategy is getting the survey to the respondent; for example, if a postcard survey is lost in the mail, that loss already results in one nonrespondent. The second part is presenting the survey in a way that promotes acknowledgment of receipt and convincing potential respondents to complete the survey. Although this point may sound obvious, it is no easy feat in the current era of information overload, in which up to 10% of people will not even realize they received a survey. [1]

Survey Medium

Surveys can be distributed by paper post (snail mail), paper in-person, e-mail/web, mobile app, audience response systems, or an interviewer (phone or in-person). Approximately half of surveys in health professions education research are distributed electronically, and fewer than 5% use a combination of mediums. [2] Table 11 summarizes the pros, cons, and practical considerations for each medium.

Some of the mediums' cons can be mitigated. Table 12 lists some popular options for scanning paper surveys to reduce the time to input results. All options involve an investment and may be best purchased by a school or department for many users to defray the cost to individuals. Table 13 lists popular programs for online surveys. Many others exist, and it may require trying a few before finding the program that best fits the needs, budgets, and institutional constraints of a particular project.

> **VOICE OF EXPERIENCE**
>
> Distributing a survey by social media and asking people to send to their friends (retweet, repost, etc.) is essentially a snowballing technique that is sometimes intentionally used when recruiting is difficult; however, this approach has important generalizability limitations and prevents calculation of a true response rate because there is no way of knowing how many people were actually invited to participate.

TABLE 11 ■ Mediums for Survey Delivery

Medium	Pros	Cons	Practical Notes
Paper post[4,9]	Hard copy motivator. Generally yields higher response rates than electronic mediums (including among younger respondents). Easy to reach large sampling frames. Visual information can help illustrate questions unlikely to be easily answered on the telephone (e.g., when a lot of quantitative [numeric] detail is required).	Usually more expensive and time-consuming than electronic (especially time-consuming data transcription to electronic format for analysis). May be lost in postal mail or not seen for months in interoffice mailbox.	Use a scanning program to streamline data transcription to electronic format for large or multi-institution sampling frames. Consider directly placing in internal mailboxes to reduce cost and risk of loss in the postal mail. Provide a pre-addressed, stamped return envelope.
Paper in-person	Hard copy motivator. Guaranteed delivery. Anecdotally the highest response rates but no empirical evidence to date.	More expensive and time consuming than electronic. Some institutional review boards may not allow physical presence of investigator, especially if investigator is in a position of power (e.g., faculty member administering survey to medical students).	Good option for sampling frames that are entire groups or classes that have a required physical meeting (e.g., required medical school class or morning report).
Electronic: web/ e-mail[5,10]	Requires fewest resources. Usually least expensive. Best and easiest format to convey pictures and graphics, as well as survey logic and item branching.	Easily ignored or inadvertently missed. Some respondents may not be electronically literate or have access.	Will be accessed by various types of electronic devices, so check that the survey appears correctly on mobile devices.
Electronic: mobile app[5]	Well formatted for mobile devices that many potential respondents have. Can send reminders that appear from the app.	Inaccessible on desktop devices. High initial cost to create (both time and money). Respondents must be willing to download app.	Consider creating for ongoing projects or if a specific sampling frame will be frequently surveyed (e.g., longitudinal surveys of medical school class).
Audience response system (ARS)[11]	Forces inclusion/ exclusion criteria because only those present can participate. Real-time data.	Forces inclusion/ exclusion criteria because only those present can participate. Not all systems export data to spreadsheet format.	Can be useful to gather data as an adjunct medium for data collection.

TABLE 11 ■ **Mediums for Survey Delivery (cont.)**

Medium	Pros	Cons	Practical Notes
In-person (phone/ Internet or interview)[12]	Very effective at limiting item nonresponse. May obtain more narrative response. Relatively high response rates. High-quality data; interviewers can probe for more complete answers and undertake validation checks at time of interview. With interviewer present to answer queries, more complex questions can be asked. Avoids need for complex item-skipping instructions based on prior answers.	The most resource-intense (time and money) option. Narrative responses must be transcribed. Risk of interviewer bias (e.g., poor training, interviewer appearance, gender, age, ethnicity, tone of voice etc.).	More commonly used in general population surveys, such as street corners or calling telephone numbers for political polling.

Paper surveys have been repeatedly shown to have the highest response rate when comparing mailed paper to Internet surveys, even among respondents in their early 20s.[3-5] No evidence to date has clearly compared in-person paper surveys, such as a survey handed out to a classroom of potential respondents, vs. mail or Internet surveys, but anecdotally, personally handing out surveys directly to a captive audience and giving them time to complete the survey tends to garner the highest response rates.

More important than the medium itself is the notion that survey designers should strongly consider employing more than one medium. Studies show that combining postal and electronic mail surveys yields better response rates than postal or electronic alone (a 7.6% absolute increase in one study), even in the current electronic culture pervasive among young adults.[3,4]

Although incremental gains may be achieved by adding mediums, two mediums should suffice[6] and should be chosen based on the characteristics specific to that particular study's sampling frame. For example, up to 98% of senior medical students use smartphones in Canada, so electronic delivery may be very effective in that group.[7] Similarly, in-person paper surveys with follow-up electronic surveys work well when the sampling frame is a well-circumscribed group, like a class, committee, or council. For example, if the sampling frame is first-year medical students, handing out the survey at a classwide assembly ensures that many of the potential respondents are immediately accessible, and a follow-up electronic survey can reach those who were absent. It is important to note that the increase in response rates from using two mediums comes from the full survey being provided in two mediums, not just from a reminder to complete the survey sent in an alternative medium, such as a postcard that instructs people to go online.[8]

Regardless of the mediums used, the survey items must be worded and presented as similarly as possible (although an identical layout is all but impossible on mobile devices) to reduce confounders, and survey designers should evaluate during data analysis whether the particular medium influenced responses. For example, a study of vaccination practices among

TABLE 12 ■ Programs That Scan Paper Surveys for Direct Import Into Statistics Programs

Service	Reads Handwriting	Pros	Cons	Pricing	Resource
IBM SPSS Data Collection Paper	No	Integrated with SPSS.	Complicated array of multiple programs. Steep learning curve.	Annual license, varying rates for commercial, academic, and personal use.	http://www.spss.com.hk/software/data-collection/paper/index.htm
Remark	No	Exports to many platforms including Excel and SPSS. Good for individuals.	Requires OMR ("fill in the bubble") design.	US $995 perpetual individual license.	https://remarksoftware.com/products/office-omr/
AutoData	Yes	Combination survey creator and text reader, including paper and electronic data incorporation.	Must use their survey creator.	Annual license, varying rates for university and commercial purchase.	http://autodata.com
Snap Surveys	No	Creates online and paper surveys. Also offers consulting services.	Must use their survey creator.	Annual individual US $2,395. Perpetual individual US $3,995.	https://www.snapsurveys.com/survey-software/paper-surveys/
Survey Pro	No	Designed for multimedia surveys.	Limited design options. Must purchase a different OMR software from Remark to scan.	US $1,295 perpetual individual.	http://www.apian.com/software/surveypro/
Survey Tracker Plus	No	Relatively inexpensive if an institution already has the Scantron scanner.	Requires Scantron scanner.	Varies with institutional annual licenses.	https://www.scantron.com/assessment-solutions/surveys/online-paper-survey-management-survey-tracker-plus/

All of these programs use an optical mark recognition (OMR) technology, but not all include the ability to convert handwriting to digital text; those that do not read handwriting require use of a third-party software.

TABLE 13 ■ Electronic Survey Options

Service	Pros	Cons	Pricing
Web-based			
Qualtrics	Academic centers often offer free to faculty. Extensive flexibility in layout and question formatting. Exports to multiple statistics programs.	Expensive, essentially requires institutional license.	Basic features: free. Full version: varies by institutional agreements.
Survey Monkey	Academic centers often offer free to faculty.	Limited visual display flexibility. Exports to .csv file with paid subscription.	<10 items, unlimited surveys: free. Additional packages: US $37–99/month.
Google Forms	Always free.	Item order in survey does not always track column order in Google Sheets. Very limited visual display and branching flexibility.	Free.
LimeSurvey	Free. Open access.	Requires computer programming knowledge.	Free.
App-based			
QuickTapSurvey	Works without Internet. Best suited for in-person surveys with an investigator.	User must have the app.	Basic: US $16 monthly individual. Additional packages: US $41–84 monthly individual.

pediatricians found significantly different responses between electronic and paper surveys because older physicians tended to reply via the paper survey, whereas younger physicians tended to reply via the electronic survey. Using two mediums can thus introduce bias not only by interaction between the respondent and the medium itself but also by some respondents specifically choosing to use a particular medium (such as older respondents preferentially choosing the paper medium).[3]

➡ VOICE OF EXPERIENCE

Consider using a scanning program that will directly import findings into a statistics program for paper surveys if the sampling frame is large (see Table 12). Some programs also feature electronic survey creation, and some are part of larger statistics packages.

➡ VOICE OF EXPERIENCE

Ensure ahead of time that the electronic survey service will deliver the results in spreadsheet format so you can formally analyze responses. Many programs, especially free versions, offer only summary statistics that prevent survey designers from looking for associations between responses that may be important to the survey question(s).

Decision to Participate

Delivery strategy also includes using adjunct methods that facilitate acknowledgment of receiving the survey and encourage the decision to participate.

Internet surveys should optimally address the individual by name, have a short and clear subject heading, and preferably be sent by someone the potential respondents already know. Postal surveys should optimally have personalized address labels, be from someone the potential respondents already know, and have text or a logo on the envelope somewhere identifying it as a survey.

The rest of the strategy is all about convincing the potential respondent to complete the survey. It is worth noting, however, that some factors influencing the decision to respond are outside of survey designers' control, namely potential respondents' gender (men are generally more likely to respond earlier),[13,14] topic salience (more likely to respond if the survey topic is of personal interest to the potential respondent),[15] and interviewers (more experienced interviewers are better, for various reasons, at convincing people to participate).[14,16,17] The best approaches to these factors are ensuring multiple invitations to gather more female responses, describe the survey well to entice more people, and hire experienced interviewers if the survey is sampling the general population in person or by phone.

The factors that are more within survey designers' influence are summarized in Table 14 and are essentially an exercise in psychology of persuasion.

Incentives are among the most commonly known and employed techniques and warrant extra discussion, although it is worth noting that incentives do not influence the decision to respond as much as survey length does (Table 14). That said, when it comes to incentives, money talks. There is no substitute for cold, hard cash in hand, despite our e-commerce and online survey society. The most evidence-based approach is between US $2.00 and US $50.00 in cash presented *up front*, *without conditions*, and in the same envelope as the survey, based on research of the general population and health professionals.[18–21]

VOICE OF EXPERIENCE

The range down to US $2.00 comes from a decades-old practice (that continues today) of sending US $2.00 bills because they are thought to include an intangible value beyond what the survey designer must pay for them because of cultural lore and their relatively uncommon status. They are still in production by the U.S. Treasury, are available at most banks, and in fact have their own award-winning documentary: www.2dollarbillmovie.com. The US $2.00 bill is a remarkably effective incentive, even among physicians with relatively high annual incomes.

Amounts for physicians, generally a less responsive cohort than other health professionals,[22] have ranged greatly, and a US $5.00 bill is probably the most reasonable number for attending physicians whereas a US $2.00 bill is probably sufficient for students and trainees. One study compared a US $2.00 bill versus a US $5.00 bill and found higher response rates for the US $5.00 bill among primary care physicians (attendings).[20] Another study looked at US $20.00 versus US $50.00 for colorectal surgeons and found a similar increase in response rate for the US $50.00.[23] A meta-analysis of the general population in several countries showed decreasing returns on investment after just US $0.50 but also showed continued significantly higher response rates up to US $5.00.[24] There is currently no evidence for a specific amount for residents, registrars, or students.[6]

Lotteries are not as effective as up-front money and, depending on the size of the sampling frame and compensation, not as cost-effective in the physician community and general population.[24–28] Therefore, the common tactic of promising "inclusion in a drawing if you take my survey" tends to be an ineffective way to improve response rates.

The compensation optimally should also be given up front, unconditionally (i.e., *not* contingent on survey completion).[19,23,24,29,30] In our experience this technique tends to be a difficult

TABLE 14 ■ **Adjunct Delivery Methods**

Strategy	Recommendation	Notes	Potential Gain
Incentives[19,20,22-24]	Give cash (or gift card) unconditionally (preferably paper survey).	Online unconditional incentives are more cumbersome. Try to include a postal version if possible.	19%
Length[13,24,33]	Advertise as "short," rather than a specific length of time. >1000 words of content decreases responses.	Different people have different interpretations of how much time is "short," so advertising "short" rather than a specific amount of time that potential respondents may interpret as "long" improves response rates.	30%
Personalization[34]	Use personalized salutations and handwritten invitations.	If using automated salutations, customize to appear more natural, such as "Dear Dr. Doe" rather than "Dear John William Doe."	9%
Authority[24]	No recommendation. Authority figures are losing effectiveness in the general population, but medicine's hierarchy may still support it.	Be sure the institutional review board approves an authority figure directly administering the survey if taking the authority figure approach.	N/A
Number of attempts[35]	Three attempts (at least).	Decreasing return on investment after three attempts. 90% of those who will respond do so within 2 weeks. Use different mediums for reminders (e.g., e-mails and post).	17%
Invitation timing[24,36,37]	No recommendation for specific day/time. Send initial invitation and reminders on different days at different times.	Invitation timing is very dependent on the characteristics of the sampling frame. Ensure there is not an exam or major group event (e.g., final exams for preclinical students) at the same time as the survey period.	N/A
Prenotification letters[12,24]	Generally helpful. Plan for it to arrive a few days before the initial invitation.	Helpful in research of public surveys but mixed evidence in health professional education (HPE) research. Is a good use of free e-mail contacts.	N/A

Potential gain in response rate given as maximum reported absolute percentage. It is important to recognize that the potential gains are not necessarily additive in actual practice because real-world human behavior can be influenced by many confounders. Some strategies do not include a percent potential gain because studies presented odds ratios in regressions, or there is insufficient evidence in the HPE population.

practice for survey designers to adopt because it can feel like throwing away money to people who will never return a survey, but placing compensation in potential respondents' hands with the survey pushes a "quid pro quo" exchange; respondents feel compelled to take the survey because they are taking the money. Convincing people to take a survey with a financial incentive is best viewed as a social exchange rather than financial exchange; US $2.00 is not a fair financial trade for most people's income. It is the social exchange that makes it work, and it has been shown repeatedly in various populations to be very effective.[1]

Finally, cash or gift card incentives work better than objects such as food or books. Often, items may not make any difference at all.[8,19] In addition, we recommend cash over gift cards, although there is limited evidence for that recommendation. One study demonstrated a 33% absolute increase in response rate for a US $25.00 check over a US $25.00 gift card among physicians.[31]

Other strategies beyond incentives are also very helpful. Multiple attempts can eventually convince people to take a survey, as can personalizing the invitation. At least three invitations are recommended (see Table 14).

VOICE OF EXPERIENCE

Lotteries are used with high frequency in HPE surveys, despite strong evidence that they are inferior to up-front, unconditional cash.

Overall, the most effective delivery strategy is one that is tailored to the way people in the sampling frame receive their most important information (usually e-mail and/or postal service) and includes a prenotification (potentially from an authority figure) followed by a short survey with at least three invitations, the first of which comes with an unconditional cash incentive. Gore-Felton and colleagues published an example of a mail survey that uses multiple strategies listed earlier.[32]

Selecting Options

Although the aforementioned recommendations paint a general approach for the best way to obtain responses, each survey must be evaluated for its own characteristics, and the **Book Introduction** example illustrates this principle well because it is a sensitive topic. First, a one-to-one encounter removes privacy and anonymity that a potential respondent may want because of the social stigma associated with substance abuse. This probably would apply to paper surveys handed out in a group setting and might lead potential participants not to respond or to provide invalid answers because they are in public. A postal paper survey followed by electronic is probably best for the example case. Additionally, there is high risk for nonresponse bias in such a sensitive survey, so the goal is not just a high response rate, but a high response rate from people who have characteristics of the areas of interest. Thus, making the survey especially salient for those with a history of substance abuse is important. If the goal of the survey, as mentioned in **Step 3: Establishing Evidence**, is to identify gaps in social support, this goal should be highlighted in the survey invitations because it directly affects individuals with substance abuse concerns.

Survey Delivery Checklist

☐ Choose 2 delivery mediums based on qualities specific to the sampling frame.
  ☐ Paper in-person
  ☐ Paper postal
  ☐ Electronic/Email
  ☐ Mobile app
  ☐ Interviewer in-person
  ☐ Interviewer phone/Internet chat
☐ If paper, choose service that exports data in a format for the appropriate statistics program.
☐ Decide on strategies to improve unit response rates.
  ☐ Incentives (unconditional vs. conditional vs. lottery)
  ☐ Length (description and <1000 words)
  ☐ Personalization
  ☐ Authority figures/Institutions
  ☐ Number of attempts (at least 3)
  ☐ Invitation timing

References

1. Dillman DA, ed. *Mail and Internet Surveys*. New York: Wiley; 2000.
2. Phillips AW, Friedman B, Utrankar A, Ta A, Reddy SR, Durning SJ. Surveys of health professions trainees: prevalence, response rates and predictive factors to guide researchers. *Acad Med*. 2016;92(2):222–228.
3. Beebe TJ, Locke GR, Barnes SA, Davern ME, Anderson KJ. Mixing web and mail methods in a survey of physicians. *Health Serv Res*. 2007;42(3 p1):1219–1234. doi: 10.1111/j.1475-6773.2006.00652.x.
4. Millar MM, Dillman DA. Improving response to web and mixed-mode surveys. *Public Opin Q*. 2011;72(2):270–286.
5. Millar M, Dillman DA. Encouraging survey response via smartphones. *Surv Pract*. 2012;5(3).
6. Phillips AW, Reddy S, Durning SJ. Improving response rates and evaluating nonresponse bias in surveys: AMEE Guide No. *102*. *Med Teach*. 2016;38(3):217–228. doi: 10.3109/0142159X.2015.1105945.
7. Tran K, Morra D, Lo V, Quan SD, Abrams H, Wu RC. Medical students and personal smartphones in the clinical environment: The impact on confidentiality of personal health information and professionalism. *J Med Internet Res*. 2014;16(5):e132. doi: 10.2196/jmir.3138.
8. Cook DA, Wittich CM, Daniels WL, West CP, Harris AM, Beebe TJ. Incentive and reminder strategies to improve response rate for internet-based physician surveys: a randomized experiment. *J Med Internet Res*. 2016;18(9):e244. doi: 10.2196/jmir.6318.
9. Scott A, Jeon S-H, Joyce CM, et al. A randomised trial and economic evaluation of the effect of response mode on response rate, response bias, and item non-response in a survey of doctors. *BMC Med Res Methodol*. 2011;11(1):126. doi: 10.1186/1471-2288-11-126.
10. Lusk C, Delclos GL, Burau K, Drawhorn DD, Aday LA. Mail versus internet surveys: determinants of method of response preferences among health professionals. *Eval Health Prof*. June 2016; doi: 10.1177/0163278707300634.
11. Bunz U. Using scantron versus an audience response system for survey research: does methodology matter when measuring computer-mediated communication competence? *Comput Human Behav*. 2005;21(2):343–359. doi: 10.1016/j.chb.2004.02.009.
12. Kellerman SE, Herold J. Physician response to surveys. a review of the literature. *Am J Prev Med*. 2001;20(1):61–67.
13. McFarlane E, Olmsted MG, Murphy J, Hill CA. Nonresponse bias in a mail survey of physicians. *Eval Health Prof*. 2007;30(2):170–185.
14. Groves RM, Couper MP. Contact-level influences on cooperation in face-to-face surveys. *J Offic Stat*. 1996;12:63–83.
15. Groves RM, Singer E, Corning A. Leverage-saliency theory of survey participation. *Public Opin Q*. 2000;64:299–308.
16. Groves RM, Couper MP. Influences of householder–interviewer interactions on survey cooperation. *In Nonresponse in Household Interview Surveys*. New York: Wiley; 1998.
17. Durrant GB, Groves RM, Staetsky L, Steele F. Effects of interviewer attitudes and behaviors on refusal in household surveys. *Public Opin Q*. 2010. http://poq.oxfordjournals.org/content/early/2010/02/24/poq.nfp098.abstract
18. Badger F, Werrett J. Room for improvement? Reporting response rates and recruitment in nursing research in the past decade. *J Adv Nurs*. 2005;51(5):502–510.
19. Church AH. Estimating the effect of incentives on mail survey response rates: a meta-analysis. *Public Opin Q*. 1993;57:62–79.
20. Asch DA, Christakis NA, Ubel PA. Conducting physician mail surveys on a limited budget. A randomized trial comparing $2 bill versus $5 bill incentives. Med Care. 1998;36(1):95–99. http://journals.lww.com/lww-medicalcare/Abstract/1998/01000/Conducting_Physician_Mail_Surveys_on_a_Limited.11.aspx
21. James JM, Bolstein R. The effect of monetary incentives and follow-up mailings on the response rate and response quality in mail surveys. *Public Opin Q*. 1990;54(3):346. doi: 10.1086/269211.
22. Cho YI, Johnson TP, VanGeest JB. Enhancing surveys of health care professionals: a meta-analysis of techniques to improve response. *Eval Health Prof*. 2013;6(3):382–407. doi: 10.1177/0163278713496425.
23. Keating NL, Zaslavsky AM, Goldstein J, West DW, Ayanian JZ. Randomized trial of $20 versus $50 incentives to increase physician survey response rates. *Med Care*. 2008;46(8):878–881.

24. Edwards P. Increasing response rates to postal questionnaires: systematic review. *BMJ.* 2002;324(7347):1183–1183. doi: 10.1136/bmj.324.7347.1183.

25. Halpern SD, Kohn R, Dornbrand-Lo A, Metkus T, Asch DA, Volpp KG. Lottery-based versus fixed incentives to increase clinicians' response to surveys. *Health Serv Res.* 2011;46(5):1663–1674.

26. Robertson J, Walkom EJ. Response rates and representativeness: a lottery incentive improves physician survey return rates. *Pharmacoepidem Drug Saf.* 2005;14:571–577. doi: 10.1002/pds.1126.

27. Gajic A, Cameron D, Hurley J. The cost-effectiveness of cash versus lottery incentives for a web-based, stated-preference community survey. *Eur J Health Econ.* 2011;13(6):789–799. doi: 10.1007/s10198-011-0332-0.

28. Tamayo-Sarver JH, Baker DW. Comparison of responses to a US 2 dollar bill versus a chance to win 250 US dollars in a mail survey of emergency physicians. *Acad Emerg Med.* 2004;11(8):888–891.

29. Berry SH, Kanouse DE. Physician response to a mailed survey: an experiment in timing of payment. *Public Opin Q.* 1987;51(1):102–114. doi: 10.1086/269018.

30. Wiant K, Geisen E, Creel D, et al. Risks and rewards of using prepaid vs. postpaid incentive checks on a survey of physicians. *BMC Med Res Methodol.* 2018;18(1):160. doi: 10.1186/s12874-018-0565-z.

31. Hogan SO, LaForce M. *Incentives in Physician Surveys: an Experiment Using Gift Cards and Checks.* American Association for Public Opinion Research, Section on Survey Research Methods. Retrieved from: http://ww2.amstat.org/sections/SRMS/Proceedings/y2008/Files/hogan.pdf. 2008:4179–4184.

32. Gore-Felton C, Koopman C, Bridges E, Thoresen C, Spiegel D. An example of maximizing survey return rates: methodological issues for health professionals. *Eval Health Prof.* June 2016;doi: 10.1177/01678702025002002.

33. Jepson C, Asch DA, Hershey JC, Ubel PA. In a mailed physician survey, questionnaire length had a threshold effect on response rate. *J Clin Epidemiol.* 2005;58(1):103–105. doi: 10.1016/j.jclinepi.2004.06.004.

34. Maheux B, Legault C, Lambert J. Increasing response rates in physicians' mail surveys: an experimental study. *Am J Public Health.* 1989;79(5):638–639. doi: 10.2105/AJPH.79.5.638.

35. Willis GB, Smith T, Lee HJ. Do additional recontacts to increase response rate improve physician survey data quality? *Med Care.* 2013;51(10):945–948. doi: 10.1097/MLR.0b013e3182a5023d.

36. Heberlein TA, Baumgartner R. Factors affecting response rates to mailed questionnaires: a quantitative analysis of the published literature. *Am Sociol Rev.* 1978;43(4):447–462.

37. Experian. Quarterly email benchmark study. Experian. https://www.experian.com/innovation/thought-leadership/q4-2011-business-benchmark.jsp. Accessed December 2, 2020.

Data Analysis

Brian E. Mavis, PhD ■ Andrew W. Phillips, MD, MEd ■ Steven J. Durning, MD, PhD

Although listed as the fifth step, data analysis begins as early as the conception of the primary objective of the survey because the research question shapes the types of data to be collected. The analysis plan (specifying chosen variables and tests) should be created before any items are written. Once data are collected, they should be evaluated with a first pass for error checking, followed by a general descriptive analysis including nonresponse bias, and, finally, analysis of differences and relationships—inferential statistics. Approaches to both quantitative and qualitative analyses are briefly discussed here.

Data First Pass

DATA SOURCES

Many of the ideas outlined in this chapter apply not only to survey data but also to data from sources other than surveys, such as test scores, rating forms, observational checklists, and content rubrics developed for short- and long-answer text (narrative response) data. Qualitative text data can be obtained through any of the aforementioned methods or can be derived from documents designed for nonresearch purposes, including patient notes, letters of reference, curricula vitae, student essays, supervisor evaluations, individualized learning plans, or personal reflections. Practically speaking, the source of the data is probably not as important as the format of the data.

Data that exist on paper need to be transformed into a digital format. It is increasingly common for surveys to be administered using digital platforms that generally eliminate the need for data entry because participants' responses—the data—are stored directly in a digital format. **Step 4: Survey Delivery** provides resources for data collection.

ERROR CHECKING

The purpose of this first review of the data is to detect unexpected values that might originate from multiple sources in the data collection process: respondents, data entry, or data coding. The two steps are 1) range checking and 2) contingency checking.

Range Checking

The most basic error checking is *range checking*, which identifies responses that are outside of the valid response options, such as rating scales (e.g., an 8 reported on an item for which the response options range from 1 to 5), or expected ranges related to demographic or personal characteristics (e.g., 225 for age from a mistype or stuck computer key) or questions that together must create a valid range (e.g., effort allocations that do not sum to 100%).

> **VOICE OF EXPERIENCE**
>
> Many electronic survey programs support range limitations, such as allowing only numerical entries between certain values for age. Applying these up front at the point of response entry can reduce the number of invalid entries.

Contingency Checking

The second step of error checking is *contingency checking*. Although range checking is done question by question, contingency checking compares responses among a set of related questions. Contingency checking is essentially reading through all the data, looking for the responses to tell a story, and finding inconsistencies in that story. This process involves not checking for outliers but rather for systemic irregularities. Problems identified during this process could be the result of respondent errors, such as when respondents misread an item, such as a negatively worded item embedded in a series of positively worded items. Other common errors result from misreading the rating scale options or not attending to instructions to "Choose one" versus "Choose all that apply." Contingency checking also can be used to identify errors in survey implementation, such as questions with conditional or response-specific branching. For example, in a study of career satisfaction, early-career faculty may be presented with additional questions, whereas mid- and late-career faculty are expected to move ahead to the next section. Any respondents misreading the instructions might complete the questions intended only for early-career faculty. These types of errors are less common in web-based surveys (which can control the flow) than paper-based surveys (which cannot), although errors in the underlying skip logic still occur for web-based surveys. Without error checking, summaries of the subgroup data would include otherwise ineligible respondents.

DATA CLEANUP

Investigators need to have a consistent process for handling situations when data anomalies are identified. Ideally, specific decision rules should have been discussed by the research team prior to the implementation of the survey. However, in practice, potential data problems cannot always be anticipated, and decision rules must be developed in real time during data analysis so that recurring problems have a documented and consistently applied solution. Decision rules may be needed for handling various types of data anomalies and for handling missing data, which often results from respondents not answering one or more questions.

Although missing data may not be as serious of an issue in descriptive and pilot studies, large amounts of missing data can create important limitations in subsequent analyses, especially for multivariate analyses. There is no published convention regarding how much missing data is too much: some authors have suggested that more that 10% is likely to result in biased analyses, although a more conservative estimate suggests that problems can occur if missing data exceeds 5%.[1] "When missing values occur for reasons beyond our control, we must make assumptions about the processes that create them. These assumptions are usually untestable" (p. 149).[2] An excellent resource for investigators interested in the mysteries of missing data is available.[3] It provides insights into strategies for identifying patterns and mechanisms of missing data, which can provide feedback about respondent survey fatigue or respondent reactions to specific questions. Also discussed are computational approaches to estimating missing data points that are beyond the scope of this chapter. Table 15 provides examples of common data irregularities.

TABLE 15 ■ Suggested Decision Rules for Data Irregularities

Irregularity	Example	Recommended Solution	Comments
Two options selected	Both "helpful" and "very helpful" circled.	Count as missing data.	Bad data may be worse than missing data.
Response outside usual range	"19" written for age in survey of medical students.	First attempt to corroborate or reassess the answer (maybe the respondent really was 19). Otherwise count as missing data.	Caution should be taken to not eliminate outliers. Potential limitation of study to include in "Discussion" section.
Free text response is illegible, or meaning is unclear	"THAT was a useful experience."	Exclude comment from analysis or create a category of "indeterminant" responses for reporting purposes.	It can be difficult to accurately detect sarcasm, irony, or hyperbole in written comments.
Missing data: individual items	Individual item(s) throughout survey are left blank.	Leave missing. Analyze item without that participant.	Bootstrapping and other methods of imputation are dangerous in the setting of social science data because the reason for the missing data may affect what that data would have been (e.g., nonresponse bias).
Missing data: full page of items	Back page or centerfold pages of survey are left blank.	For nonanonymous surveys, return incomplete portions to respondent for completion. Otherwise leave missing. Analyze items without that participant.	More likely to occur in paper surveys: page numbers, booklet formats, and clear instructions can help reduce likelihood of this.
Missing data: multiple items at end of survey	Items at the end of the survey more likely to be missing than earlier items.	Leave missing. Analyze items without that participant.	Survey fatigue resulting from long surveys. Consider providing milestone messages to respondents (e.g., "Almost there... 75% done!").

(Continued)

TABLE 15 ■ Suggested Decision Rules for Data Irregularities (*cont.*)

Irregularity	Example	Recommended Solution	Comments
Missing data: one or multiple related items	Question wording or response options challenging for respondents.	Leave missing. Analyze items without that participant.	Often related to items that have challenging grammar, use of unfamiliar terms or acronyms, or vocabulary that exceeds the literacy level of respondents.
Missing data: one or multiple related items	Item or section on topics perceived as sensitive or threatening by respondents, such as illegal or socially undesirable behavior.	Leave missing. Analyze items without that participant.	It is difficult to collect information in certain content areas, particularly for nonanonymous surveys.

Every situation is different, and these are generalized suggestions that are conservative approaches that can negatively affect statistical power.

Quantitative Analysis

DATA ANALYSIS RESOURCES

Several software options for data analysis are available. Many spreadsheet applications have built-in statistical functions that can be used to generate descriptive and bivariate statistics. Microsoft Excel[5] and Google Sheets[6] provide online resources to facilitate analyses. There also are specialized statistical software packages designed specifically for quantitative analyses, including R, SAS, STATA, and SPSS, that large and complex data sets might require. Similarly, a number of software packages are available to facilitate qualitative analyses of textual data, including Atlas.ti, Dedoose, and NVivo. A less expensive alternative for narrative responses is simply printing the text and color-coding by hand with highlighters or colored pencils or doing so electronically to identify the various themes. Although seemingly arduous, this type of "analog" manual process of analyzing qualitative data is often preferred by some survey designers, especially when working with relatively small data sets. See Appendix 5 for an example with explanation.

Regardless of the software used for data analysis, the best resources are colleagues who are knowledgeable in the types of analyses and the software needed for the project. The specific analyses and program to perform them should be established during the item-writing process (see **Step 2: Survey Construction**) to ensure that items are formatted correctly for the proposed analyses. The good news is that many survey studies do not require expensive software or equipment. However, for studies that require more complex analyses, it is prudent to consider adding someone knowledgeable about anticipated data analysis needs early when developing the research team (e.g., a psychometrician or statistician).

 VOICE OF EXPERIENCE

Pilot test your analyses by performing a complete data analysis on the pilot data collected, using the same statistical tests and the same computer software that will be used on the actual data set. Sometimes survey creation tools export data in unexpected ways that are incompatible with the planned analysis, such as "Check all that apply" exporting only boxes that were checked, so it is impossible to know whether unchecked boxes represent "No" or a skipped item.

TYPES OF MEASUREMENTS

It is very important to understand the types of variables and the levels of measurement they represent. Most statistics textbooks identify four levels of measurement:[7]

- *nominal:* variables that do not have any intrinsic numeric value; values function as names or labels. Examples include Sex (1 = male; 2 = female); Mentor Group (1 = Wagner, 2 = Malinowski, 3 = Chang, 4 = Stauff, 5 = Zheng, 6 = Pylman); Specialty (1 = Allergy and Immunology … 24 = Urology); State (1 = Alabama … 50 = Wyoming); etc.
- *ordinal:* variables that have an implied order, but the difference between adjacent values is uncertain or not meaningful. Examples include Academic Rank (1 = Instructor, 2 = Assistant Professor, 3 = Associate Professor, 4 = Full Professor); Level of Training (1 = Medical Student, 2 = Resident, 3 = Attending Physician); Symptom Frequency (1 = Rarely, 2 = Seldom, 3 = Sometimes, 4 = Often, 5 = Almost Always); etc.
- *interval:* variables where the values are uniform in terms of order and differences between adjacent values. Most assessments of traits, ability or knowledge are considered to be interval measures because the zero point is arbitrary rather than absolute. Any zero point that does exist is arbitrary and a result of the sampling of questions on the test. For example, someone who scores zero on a statistics test likely does have some knowledge of statistics but was unable to answer any of the questions correctly. This person's level of knowledge is not detectable by this test because of the arbitrary zero point defined by the specific questions.[8] Examples of common interval measures include test scores such as IQ, MCATs, and shelf examinations. In practice, many psychosocial constructs such as emotional intelligence, confidence, preparedness, and other personality attributes of interest to medical educators are considered to approximate interval measures.[7,8]
- *ratio:* variables have the same properties as interval variables with the addition of a true or absolute zero point. Examples include height, weight, completion time, age, number of publications, etc.

Statisticians can talk endlessly about levels of measurement, nuances among different measurement levels, and examples of exceptions to the rule. An important example is data derived from ratings scales, generally considered ordinal data. The thought is that such data cannot be interval because it is unclear if the magnitude of the difference in, for example, satisfaction from a rating of 4 = satisfied and 5 = very satisfied is the same as the difference between 2 = dissatisfied and 3 = neither satisfied nor dissatisfied. However, in practice, it is common for investigators to report means and standard deviations for rating scale data (ordinal), a property reserved for interval and ratio level measures. Further, inferential statistics comparing the satisfaction between two or more groups are commonly reported in published studies, and the decision to treat the data as ordinal or interval determines which tests are appropriate, which can affect statistical power.

There is a multitude of publications on both sides of the argument, and the take away message is that *often* it is acceptable to consider Likert-type items as interval, but *not always.*[9–11] For example, if multiple items are combined to create a scale score, then the distribution of the aggregated score is more important than distributions of the individual items. If the analysis focuses on individual items, then the distribution of responses becomes important. There are situations when respondents do not use all available response options, resulting in one or more response options being chosen by few or no respondents. In essence, what might have been designed as a five-point response scale, in practice becomes a three-point scale if respondents seldom choose the extreme values. Similarly, responses skewed to one end of a response scale present challenges. In these cases, an ordinal approach is recommended.

The most conservative approach, recommended for novice survey designers and those without guidance from statisticians, is to treat Likert-type items as ordinal data, and use statistical approaches suitable to ordinal data. If appropriate assumptions are met, however, it is reasonable to treat Likert-type items as interval data for analyses.

DESCRIPTIVE ANALYSIS

Describe the Context

All survey studies need a "Table 1" that describes demographics and contextual information about the respondents, and these findings should be the first to be analyzed. See the checklist at the end of this chapter for analyses that should be considered.

Histograms and bar charts are useful visualization tools for variables of all levels of measurement; they provide insight into the distribution of the values and are an important part of the analysis even if they are not included in the manuscript.[7] For ratio and interval variables (e.g., test scores, demographic characteristics, and budget data), descriptive statistics provide a numeric summary of the response distribution. The descriptive statistics most commonly used are *means* and *standard deviations* to represent the average and the spread around the average. Additional statistics, such as minimum and maximum values and quartiles, can be helpful as well. These descriptive statistics are particularly useful for variables that have a normal or bell-shaped distribution. If the histogram shows a distribution that is less bell-shaped or less symmetrical, the mean by itself becomes a less meaningful measure of central tendency and should be accompanied by the *median* and *mode*. As a reminder, the mean is the arithmetic average of a variable, whereas the median is the center point of the distribution or 50th percentile, and the mode is the most frequent response. The mean, median, and mode are the same for a normal distribution, but they diverge the more the distribution deviates from normal.

An internal summary document is a helpful way to organize the descriptive statistics as a master resource when writing a report or publication. One approach to this task is to use the original questionnaire as the template to organize the data summary, typing or hand-writing results alongside the questions. Whether the means, standard deviations, percentages, number of responses, etc., for each item are typed or handwritten on a copy of the original document, there will be a handy reference document that can aid in finding trends, relationships, and the general story that the data tell.

Describe the Respondents

The *response rate* is critical to reporting who responded to the survey, and a *nonresponse bias* analysis is critical to reporting whether the respondents were representative of the original target group (*sampling frame*).

The response rate is essentially the proportion of individuals who participated in a survey out of all those eligible to participate. In reality, this calculation is more complicated and depends on how "eligible" and "participated" are defined.[12,13] For example, the response rate calculation can be adjusted to include only those respondents who completed the whole survey or respondents who completed any part of the survey. The complete equation for response rate (RR) is given by

$$RR = \frac{(\text{complete surveys}) + (\text{partial surveys})}{(\text{complete} + \text{partial surveys}) + (\text{refusal} + \text{noncontact} + \text{other}) + e(\text{unknown if eligible} + \text{unknown other})} \quad [1]$$

where e is the estimated proportion of people who are actually eligible out of the group of potential respondents whose eligibility is not known (see example below). The different definitions include and exclude different parts of this large equation based on study assumptions. Fig. 4 illustrates each of the definitions.

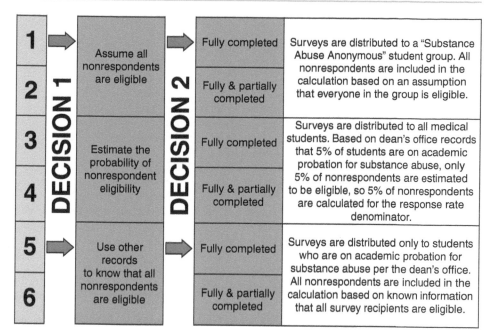

Fig. 4 How to Calculate Response Rate. Two major decisions turn into six total definitions. The first decision yields three pairs; the second decision distinguishes within the pairs. Odd number definitions only include fully completed surveys in the numerator, whereas even number definitions include fully and partially (some missing questions) completed surveys in the numerator. The example explanations refer to the running case from the **Book Introduction**.

Referring to the **Book Introduction** example, the sampling frame is students at Health Professions Education (HPE) University who have a history of substance abuse. Definitions 1, 2, 5, and 6 are similar in that the denominator is the same. Definitions 1 and 2 *assume* everyone receiving the survey is eligible (such as showing up to a Substance Abuse Anonymous meeting), whereas definitions 5 and 6 *know* everyone receiving the survey is eligible (such as being on academic probation for confirmed substance abuse). The ideal approach for the study on substance abuse described in the **Book Introduction** would probably be to distribute the survey only to those who are known to be eligible (20 students), and use definitions 5 or 6. If 10 surveys are fully completed and 5 surveys are partially completed, the response rate for definition 5 would be:

$$\frac{(10)}{(10+5)+(5)+(0)} = 0.50 = 50\% \quad [2]$$

and definition 6 would be:

$$\frac{(10)+(5)}{(10+5)+(5)+(0)} = 0.75 = 75\% \quad [3]$$

However, an ethics board or the dean's office might not allow access to those students who are on probation because of privacy concerns. But sending the survey to the entire student body with so few students eligible would decrease the response rate tremendously if all students were assumed to be eligible. That is where response rates 3 and 4 are helpful. If the dean's office releases the information that 20 students are on probation for known substance abuse, then we can estimate that 20/400 students (or 5%) are eligible and apply that number to all of the nonresponses.

Assuming the same 10 fully completed and 5 partially completed surveys, response rate definition 3 would be:

$$\frac{(10)}{(10+5)+(0)+0.05(385)} = 0.29 = 29\% \qquad [4]$$

Thus, although not perfect, definitions 3 and 4 can be helpful when eligibility status cannot be known. Without the eligibility estimate, the response rate would have been 10/400 = 2.5% and not an accurate reflection of the sampling frame. The definitions become complicated quickly if eligibility and contact success (e.g., expired emails) must be considered. It is best to read carefully through the official AAPOR definitions document.[12]

Nonresponse bias is a bias of results introduced by not achieving a representative sample from the sampling frame, and importantly, those not responding have attributes, beliefs, or experiences that interact with the survey in some way to influence results. Nonresponse bias should *always* be evaluated, regardless of response rate, because response rate accounts for only approximately 10% of variance in nonresponse bias. It is not just how many people did not respond, but, more importantly, *why* they did not respond that creates nonresponse bias. For example, a survey about addiction may have a 90% response rate but nonetheless suffer from nonresponse bias if many of the missing 10% have a relationship with addiction.[14]

VOICE OF EXPERIENCE

A high response rate does not imply that the survey is free of nonresponse bias, and a low response rate does not imply that the survey suffers from nonresponse bias. The response rate contributes a mere 10% of the variance in nonresponse bias. Therefore, the actual nonresponse bias should always be directly assessed.

Capturing nonresponse bias is essentially a Schrödinger's cat scenario because if the survey designer captures data from a nonrespondent, the person becomes, by definition, a respondent. If the person remains a nonrespondent, the survey designer can only use alternative data. Thus, the two main families of evaluating nonresponse bias are using proxy data and using proxy non-respondents. Because of the limitations of both methods, we recommend using one of each, although there are no formal guidelines. Fig. 5 shows a simple approach[15] for each, using the **Book Introduction** example; however, many more options exist.[16] If nonresponse bias is present, the data may need to be weighted, which adjusts the sample to more accurately reflect characteristics of the population. This weighting is best handled by an experienced statistician.

ANSWER THE RESEARCH QUESTION(S)

Ideally, the original study design included a plan for analysis; the research questions that guide the study also guide analysis and reporting. The research questions can help focus survey design and help limit extraneous questions not directly related to the purpose of the study. An analysis plan such as the one described in **Step 1: Needs Assessment** can also reduce the risk of data dredging, which refers to the practice of conducting too many analyses, such that something statistically significant eventually emerges but most likely as a result of chance rather than a meaningful relationship. The research questions provide boundaries for the analyses and help the research team focus amid what might seem like "tons of data." Research questions also can help avoid such fishing expeditions. Good research questions have helpful words:

Describe learner satisfaction…
Compare the career interests of science and nonscience majors …
Estimate the association between confidence and age…
Predict USMLE Step 1 performance based on …

Proxy Nonrespondent

Use true respondents who are similar to nonrespondents to be proxy nonrespondents.

RESPONDENTS	vs	NONRESPONDENTS
Actual respondent		Proxy nonrespondent
Actual data		Actual data

Nonresponse bias can be quantitatively determined by:

$$NRB = (\%_{nonrespondents}) \times [(mean_{actualrespondents}) - (mean_{proxynonrespondents})]$$

Wave analysis uses results from the last wave of respondents as data from proxy nonrespondents under the assumption that whatever factors contributed to people responding late may also be factors that contributed to people not responding at all. The first wave can be defined as responses received between initial and second invitations; the last wave can be defined as responses received between last invitation and close of survey.

Practical Application

1) Select which item(s) to compare (reflective of the overall instrument)
2) Apply nonresponse bias equation
3) IF practically significant, discuss weighting data with statistician

Suppose the mean of a representative item with a 5 point scale is 3.0 for the first wave and 2.5 for the last wave of respondents. Further assume a response rate of 60%, any definition.

1) Use Question X as a representative item
2) Nonresponse bias = (%nonrespondents) X [(mean_proxynonrespondents) – (mean_proxynonrespondents)]
   ➤ NRB = 0.4 x [(3)-(2.5)]
   ➤ NRB = 0.4 x [0.5]
   ➤ NRB = 0.2
3) 0.2 on a 5 point scale is a 4% difference seen in the nonrespondents, unlikely to have practical significance and so likely does not need to be weighted. The decision of practical significance is up to the researchers.

Proxy Data

Use known data about the nonrespondents (or entire population) to be proxy survey data.

RESPONDENTS	vs	NONRESPONDENTS
Actual respondent		Actual nonrespondent
Actual data		Proxy data

Nonresponse bias cannot be quantitatively determined with proxy data. Instead, known data about the population or—if possible—the nonrespondents specifically is used.

Demographic information between respondents and the population or the nonrespondents is commonly used. The variable(s) tested should be pertinent to the study. Examples include age, sex, gender, ethnicity, exam scores, etc.

Practical Application

1) Select which demographics to compare (preferably have theoretical relationship)
2) Apply statistical tests as appropriate for data type(s)
3) IF statistically significant and IF practically significant, discuss weighting data with statistician

Suppose 40% of the 15 respondents are male, and the sampling frame of 20 people is known to be 50% male.

1) Compare % males since there is a known relationship between males and substance abuse
2) 6 of 15 respondents (40%) reported being male vs 10 of 20 people (50%) in the sampling frame are known to be male from dean's office records
   ➤ $X2(1)=2.4$, p=.121
3) Despite a theoretical relationship between male gender and substance abuse, there is not a statistically significant difference in respondents' gender. If the difference had been significant, a statistician would need to be consulted to weight the responses by gender.

Fig. 5 Two Methods of Calculating Nonresponse Bias. Refer to the **Book Introduction** for the example case specifics.

The specific question drives the appropriate statistical test. For example, "Estimate the association between confidence and age..." likely requires a Spearman's or Pearson's correlation coefficient. Indications and assumptions for the various tests are beyond the scope of this text, but it is worth emphasizing that the approach to the data should always center around the original research question(s). We recommend an analysis plan as part of the initial survey instrument development such as Appendix 1.

Analysis of Survey Items

The validity and reliability of the survey scores must be analyzed, even if the instrument has prior validity evidence. Specifics about validity and reliability are described in **Step 3: Establishing Evidence**, but it is important to recognize that the analysis of the item scores has little meaning if the analysis of the scale scores or other measures is not performed and deemed sufficient.

Just as with the contextual data (e.g., demographics), all instrument items, domains, and scales (as applicable to the study) should be analyzed (see **Step 3: Establishing Evidence**) with basic descriptions such as mean and standard deviation (or median and mode), 95% confidence interval, and skew and kurtosis. It is advisable to make a histogram as well. That is not to say that all of these analyses must be reported, but they should be performed for internal review.

Analyzing Items vs. Domains vs. Scales

Many standardized questionnaires have been developed to measure attitudes, beliefs, and psychological characteristics. These questionnaire items create domains, and the domains create an overall scale. Which parts to analyze (items vs. domains vs. scales) depends on the questions built in **Step 1: Needs Assessment**. No matter the circumstances, it is not good practice to run multiple comparisons and contrasts on every item, domain, and scale.

If the primary objective involves a psychometric construct, such as burnout, the overall burnout scale score is of most interest and should be analyzed with the other data of interest (e.g., board scores, age, specialty, years of practice, etc.). If the primary or secondary objective were to stratify and explore burnout, then the subscores—emotional exhaustion, meaningfulness, and depersonalization—might be of interest. However, exploring the individual items is likely to only advance data dredging. An exception might be when a study focuses on the development of a new measure of a construct, when specific item-level analysis is important.

In contrast, some surveys do not lend themselves well to scale scores, such as those seeking opinions in which each opinion is about a topic but not necessarily a construct, or those with questions designed to elicit descriptive or factual information. Here the domain or scale results (if even possible) are not as meaningful as the individual survey items.

Combining or Collapsing Response Options: Pros, Cons, Indications

Many survey items rely on responses framed within a five-point rating scale, although these principles can apply to other types of rating scales as well. There also are situations when response options might be intentionally combined. One reason to do this is to create categories that highlight differences, such as creating a single category of *satisfaction* by combining *satisfied* and *very satisfied* responses. Another possible situation is when respondents overall avoid extreme rating options and do not use the complete range of available response options (e.g., using 2, 3, and 4 and avoiding 1 and 5 on a five-point rating scale). Recalling the example earlier, combining the *satisfied* and *very satisfied* responses together and combining the *dissatisfied* and *very dissatisfied* into another response category would create a three-category variable for analysis and reporting.

Sometimes it can be helpful to reduce multiple points to a dichotomous variable as well, whether because the relationship is more clearly presented that way, there is greater statistical power with fewer variables, or some other reason. For example, responses designed to elicit frequency of an event (1 = Never, 2 = Once, 3 = Twice, 4 = Three or more times) can be combined to create a dichotomous variable indicating the event occurred (combining 2, 3, and 4) or did not occur (1 = Never).

It is imperative to report, whether in the "Methods" or "Results" section, that a scale was condensed, and it is a good idea for the sake of transparency to have the original, full-version scale data available in an appendix.

Difficult Formats

"Select all that apply" essentially creates a series of binary items within a single survey question, which makes analysis difficult. Each response option must be analyzed as a unique binary item, and the binary nature makes associations more difficult to assess. For example, associations cannot be assessed, even though there may be a relationship, because all of the options are part of the same survey question. There is also some evidence that "Check all that apply" items can encourage respondents to be less thoughtful in their responses (i.e., to satisfice). Thus other formats, such as "Check yes or no" with a series of options (rather than "Select all that apply"), should be explored earlier in the design phase (see **Step 2: Survey Construction**).

Free text "other" response options are sometimes included in items such as those seeking opinions, but not in scale items. The "other" category can be analyzed as simply another category in an item producing nominal data. Sometimes respondents write something in "other" that can be reasonably categorized with one of pre existing options, and recoding the response to that option may be reasonable at the discretion of the survey designers but must be reported in the manuscript.

"No opinion" (NO) and "not applicable" (NA) response options are handled in various ways, not least of which is avoiding them altogether in the item creation phase (see **Step 2: Survey Construction**). If attached to a scale item, the NO or NA should not be analyzed as part of the interval or ordinal scale, but rather reported as a separate frequency. NO and NA are different from a neutral opinion on an odd-numbered scale, which would be analyzed as part of the scale. (Pros and cons to even vs odd-numbered scales are in **Step 2: Survey Construction**). Regardless, the use of NO or NA is generally discouraged unless it is absolutely necessary. Further, if a NO or NA is attached to a nominal item, the frequency of the NO or NA response may be reported just as the other nominal response options.

Narrative Response Codes

A brief explanation for analysis of narrative response items is provided later in this chapter, but those codes can also be analyzed numerically with other items. For example, a demographic answer to a gender or age question might have a relationship with narrative response options. The frequencies of each code in a narrative response option can sometimes be treated the same as frequencies for nominal response options in traditional survey items and compared as such with other items adhering to the same principles noted earlier.

Statistical Tests

The essentials of basic statistical tests are in Appendix 6. There are a number of excellent resources to guide the choice of statistical tests.[7,17,18] A survey designer with a background in statistics or a statistician should assist with even "simple" inferential statistics tests because of the complexities of assumptions and interactions of variables that may not be evident to inexperienced survey designers. The table included as Appendix 6 is provided only as a quick reference tool and is not a substitute for a full understanding of each of the tests.

Regardless of which specific tests are used, statistical significance will be part of the analysis. Statistical significance refers to the likelihood that a relationship among variables did not occur by chance. If the same study is conducted a hundred times, how many times would this result be obtained? Less common findings are considered less likely the result of chance and more likely indicative of genuine relationships among variables, resulting from experience, intervention, or other factors. How rare does a result have to be to be considered statistically significant? In general, results that would be expected less than 5% of the time by chance are described as statistically significant, and this is represented as $p < 0.05$. When a statistical test yields a result that has a p-value < 0.05, the finding is considered significant. If the p-value is equal to or greater than 0.05 ($p \geq 0.05$), then the finding is not statistically significant. There are situations when other p-values might be considered. When multiple statistical tests are used, the p-value can be corrected for multiple comparisons, generally resulting in a lower (more stringent) p-value threshold. This is referred to as the familywise error rate.[7] In contrast, an investigator might use a less stringent criterion such as $p < 0.10$ for an exploratory study, particularly if the sample size is limited. This practice is controversial insofar as its application defies the intention behind the use of a 5% probability level as a dichotomous standard for determining statistical significance.

The standard of 5% as the determination of statistical significance is an arbitrary but generally accepted criterion for interpreting analyses.[7,17] The use of $p < 0.05$ is ubiquitous and remains a standard of statistical practice. Nonetheless, there is a continuing debate about the use, abuse, and misinterpretation of statistical significance tests that is far beyond the scope of this chapter but is nonetheless interesting reading.[19-21]

Confidence Intervals

Like the discussion of p-value, the concept of confidence interval is probability based. Studies are based on samples from a population of eligible participants, and when summary statistics such as means or proportions are calculated, they are based on the data derived from the sample. If the mean emotional intelligence of a sample of medical students were measured at 110 using an assessment tool, would we get the same mean if another sample of medical students participated in the study? If the study were replicated on 100 samples, how much would the mean emotional intelligence vary across 100 replications? A confidence interval is a range that is likely to contain the true value of the population mean. Confidence intervals are usually estimated for 95% certainty, representing an upper and lower bound for the true value, such as *there is 95% probability that the mean emotional intelligence is between 107 and 113*. Calculation of the confidence interval is based on the size and variability of the sample. The 95% confidence interval is generated by software applications that include statistical analysis and can also be calculated by hand.[7,17]

Effect Size

Statistical significance provides an indication of whether or not the observed relationship among variables is unlikely by chance and therefore possibly true. It is increasingly common to report effect sizes in addition to statistical significance as a useful metric for understanding the magnitude of relationships among variables, which is also known as the practical significance of the findings.[7] The larger the effect size, the larger the relationship among variables. Although a probability analysis might identify a statistically significant relationship, it is the effect size that communicates the usefulness or meaningfulness of the relationship. There are multiple resources for guidance on how to calculate effect size (e.g., Cohen[22] or Sullivan and Feinn[23]).

 VOICE OF EXPERIENCE

Whether or not to provide p-value or confidence interval and whether to include effect size is a property of the statistical test, not the data source. As practical advice, we recommend running the analysis for all three and including them in the internal results document because each provides different insights into the data. Several HPE journals now provide instructions to authors specifically indicating which values are expected, and those instructions should be followed. Having all numbers available makes it easier to meet any journal's requirements.

Qualitative Analysis

DATA VARIETY

Another important aspect of survey data is the analysis of narrative survey responses. This task can vary considerably in terms of time and effort depending on the specificity of the survey question. Sometimes the responses are only a few words, such as prompts to enter specific information after choosing "Other" from a list of options. At the other extreme, surveys can include unbounded text boxes that provide respondents the opportunity to write a paragraph outlining strengths and weaknesses of their educational experience. In practice, most text responses are somewhere in between. For example, when asked "What are the strengths of this instructor?" the responses are likely to address a range of issues related to teaching skills, interpersonal and facilitation skills, content knowledge, preparedness, assessment, feedback, etc. Less focused questions (e.g., What did you learn from this course?) could generate a broad range of responses that go beyond the objectives listed in the syllabus and require thoughtful categorization to yield meaningful results.

APPROACH TO QUALITATIVE SURVEY DATA

It is important to note that qualitative data analysis is a field unto itself, and a survey is not a substitute for the time-intensive process of a full and proper qualitative study and the rich data it yields.[24] The narrative response options in surveys should be limited in scope and number. Qualitative analysis represents a broad field of methodologies, such as thematic analysis, discourse analysis, and phenomenological analysis.[25] For survey-based data, thematic analysis is the most commonly used analytic approach. In this chapter, we describe a general set of procedures that can be applied to most survey text data. There are two approaches to analyzing qualitative survey data, depending on whether there is a predefined list of likely responses or whether the goal is to unpack emergent themes without prior expectations or definitions.

THEMATIC SUMMARY

A preexisting list of likely responses can be used to create a rubric for guiding the categorization of responses. Questions that have finite boundaries or where the number of possible open-ended responses is limited are ideal. Examples include likely differential diagnoses in the context of a specific case, use of self-directed learning strategies, or Systems Engineering Initiative for Patient Safety (SEIPS) elements. Defining the set of likely responses might require reviewing relevant curricular content or study resources, consultation with colleagues, and/or pilot testing the question to determine the probable responses.

If the goal is to create a thematic summary of responses, the approach is more inductive,[25] and thematic development is an iterative process. The first step is reading the text responses and making note of the themes that emerge. While reading, it might become apparent that some themes have subcategories (subthemes) that can be meaningful in reporting the survey results: for example, comments about learner assessment could focus on content, quality, frequency, or feedback.

If the number of responses is large, it might not be necessary to read all of them to develop the list of themes for categorizing responses. With continued reading it is possible to reach a point when no new categories emerge, in which case saturation has been achieved, and it is likely that the list of themes can be used to categorize most if not all the text comments. It is important not to lose sight of the purpose of the survey; consider the emerging themes in terms of the survey purpose and the specific question that prompted the responses. At this point it is good practice to have others review the list of themes to ensure that the content has been reliably mapped and the logic of categories makes sense to others.

Next is pilot testing the coding system. For the pilot test, all coders independently categorize a common set of responses and afterward compare their categorizations. Discussing differences of interpretation and nuance provides an opportunity for coders to develop a common mental framework for their work and reduces ambiguities of category definitions, thereby enhancing the coding system. When there is confidence that the coding system can be reliably used by multiple coders, analysis of the data can begin. If the discussion of the initial coded text responses resulted in multiple changes to the category system, a second pilot test can be useful to confirm the reliability of the coders.

Coding the text is itself an iterative process. The analysis of test responses involves a process of constant comparison.[26] Categories themselves are refined through the coding process as new text examples are considered in the context of prior coded examples in terms of similarity.

Seemingly discrepant examples are compared with ideal examples to aid defining the boundaries of what is included within a specific category.[27] The use of the constant comparison method and discrepant case analysis during the coding process frequently results in thematic categories being reorganized, renamed or redefined.[28] These changes result in categorization schemes that more meaningfully represent the experiences of respondents. As the category system evolves, recoding of earlier material is necessary.

Because a single response could receive multiple codes, the number of codes will likely exceed the number of respondents and will total to more than 100%. The frequencies of the codes can be reported for the sample overall and for subgroups of respondents and treated like nominal data, as described earlier.

PRACTICAL CONSIDERATIONS

A number of software applications have been developed to read text files and help code them according to specific criteria. Most often this is accomplished by simple word counts, which can be useful for comparing text to a user-defined dictionary of words, such as key concepts or words representing either positive or negative emotions.

Significant challenges when analyzing narrative responses are the time and resources required. Because of this, survey designers should be thoughtful about the number of narrative response questions and the crafting of the questions to elicit the desired information.

Another common challenge occurs during thematic analysis and code development. It can be difficult to be objective when reading the narrative responses. Having someone less closely affiliated with the study and data collection can be one approach to maintain objectivity. Another approach would be to code in pairs: either both investigators coding all responses twice or periodically comparing the coding of a common set of responses. Cohen's kappa is commonly used to evaluate interrater reliability of codes. A subset of responses and their codes is usually analyzed in full qualitative studies, but because survey qualitative items should be relatively small in scope and frequency, analyzing all responses and codes may also be reasonable. Sometimes initial coding is not reliable or does not provide meaningful results and must be reanalyzed. If this occurs, it should be mentioned in the manuscript.

Data Analysis Checklist

- ☐ Perform a first pass of the data.
    - ☐ Range and contingency checking
    - ☐ Consistent process for data anomalies
- ☐ Establish levels of measurement for the data.
- ☐ Provide a descriptive analysis.
    - ☐ "Table 1" of demographics and baseline participant characteristics
    - ☐ Response rate
    - ☐ Nonresponse bias assessment
- ☐ Answer the research question.
    - ☐ Descriptive analyses of items, domains, and/or scales depending on study objectives
    - ☐ Inferential statistics
- ☐ Evaluate qualitative data if applicable.

References

1. Dong Y, Peng CYJ. Principled missing data analysis methods for researchers. *SpringerPlus*. 2013;2(1):222. doi:10.1186/2193-1801-2-222.
2. Schafer JL, Graham JW. Missing data: our view of the state of the art. *Psychol Methods*. 2002;7(2): 147–177.
3. Enders CK. *Applied Missing Data Analysis*. New York: Guilford Press; 2010.
4. Anderson JV, Mavis BE, Robison JI, Stöffelmayr BE. A worksite weight management program to reinforce behavior. *J Occup Med*. 1993;35(8):800–804.
5. Microsoft Office: Statistical Functions for Excel. https://support.office.com/en-us/article/statistical-functions-reference-624dac86-a375-4435-bc25-76d659719ffd. Accessed February 6, 2020.
6. Google Sheets Function List. https://support.google.com/docs/table/25273?hl=en. Accessed February 6, 2020.
7. Norman GR, Streiner DL. *Biostatistics: The Bare Essentials*. 4th ed. Shelton, CT: People's Medical Publishing House; 2014.
8. Ghiselli EE, Campbell JP, Zedeck S. *Measurement Theory for the Behavioral Sciences*. New York: WH Freeman and Company; 1981.
9. Jamieson S. Likert scales: how to (ab)use them. *Med Educ*. 2004;38:1212–1218.
10. Norman G, Likert scales: levels of measurement and the "laws" of statistics. *Adv Health Sci Educ*. 2010;15(5):625–632.
11. Joshi A, Kale S, Chandel S, Pal DK. Likert scale: explored and explained. *Br J Appl Sci Technol*. 2015;7(4):396–403.
12. The American Association for Public Opinion Research. Standard Definitions: Final Dispositions of Case Codes and Outcome Rates for Surveys. 9th edition. AAPOR. Available from: https://www.aapor.org/AAPOR_Main/media/publications/Standard-Definitions20169theditionfinal.pdf. Accessed February 6, 2020.
13. Phillips AW, Friedman B, Durning SJ. How to calculate a survey response rate: best practices. *Acad Med*. 2017;92(2):269.
14. Groves RM, Peytcheva E. The impact of nonresponse rates on nonresponse bias: a meta-analysis. *Public Opin Q*. 2008;72(2):167–189.
15. Phillips AW, Reddy S, Durning SJ. Improving response rates and evaluating nonresponse bias in surveys: AMEE Guide No. 102. *Med Teach*. 2016;38(3):217–228.
16. Halbesleben JR, Whitman MV. Evaluating survey quality in health services research: a decision framework for assessing nonresponse bias. *Health Serv Res*. 2013;48(3):913–930.
17. Harris M, Taylor G. *Medical Statistics Made Easy*. 3rd ed. Banbury, UK: Scion Publishing; 2014.
18. Windish DM, Deiner-West M. A clinician-educator's roadmap to choosing and interpreting statistical tests. *J Gen Intern Med*. 2006;21:656–660.
19. Lambdin C. Significance tests as sorcery: science is empirical—significance tests are not. *Theory Psychol*. 2012;22(1):67–90.
20. Greenland S, Senn SJ, Rothman KJ, Carlin JB, Poole C, Goodman SN, et al. Statistical tests, P values, confidence intervals, and power: a guide to misinterpretations. *Eur J Epidemiol*. 2016;31:337–350. 10.1007/s10654-016-0149-3.
21. Wasserstein RL, Lazar NA. The ASA Statement on p-values: context, process, and purpose. *Am Stat*. 2016;70(2):129–133. doi: 10.1080/00031305.2016.1154108.
22. Cohen J. *Statistical Power Analysis for the Behavioral Sciences*. 2nd ed. Hillsdale, NJ: Lawrence Erlbaum Associates; 1988.
23. Sullivan GM, Feinn R. Using effect size—or why the p value is not enough. *J Grad Med Educ*. 2012;4(3):279–282.
24. LaDonna KA, Taylor T, Lingard L. Why open-ended survey questions are unlikely to support rigorous qualitative insights. *Acad Med*. 2018;93(3):347–349.
25. Kalpokaite N, Radivojevic I. Demystifying qualitative data analysis for novice qualitative researchers. *The Qualitative Report*. 2019;24(13):44–57. Retrieved from https://nsuworks.nova.edu/tqr/vol24/iss13/5. Accessed February 6, 2020.

26. Dye JF, Schatz IM, Rosenberg BA, Coleman ST. Constant comparison method: a kaleidoscope of data. *The Qualitative Report*. 2000;4(1):1–10. Retrieved from https://nsuworks.nova.edu/tqr/vol4/iss1/8. Accessed February 6, 2020.

27. Morrow SL. Quality and trustworthiness in qualitative research in counseling psychology. *J Couns Psychol*. 2005;52:250–260.

28. Kennedy TJ, Lingard LA. Making sense of grounded theory in medical education. *Med Educ*. 2006;40:101–108.

Reporting Guidelines

Anthony R. Artino, Jr., PhD ■ Anna T. Cianciolo, PhD ■ Erik W. Driessen, PhD ■ David P. Sklar, MD ■ Steven J. Durning, MD, PhD

CHAPTER OUTLINE

When designed and implemented carefully, surveys can be used to answer questions that other research methods cannot (see **Step 1: Needs Assessment**).[1] The final challenge in survey-based research is to document the study in a complete and compelling way so the survey instrument and its data are meaningful, set in the appropriate context, and potentially useful to others. Effective survey-based research reports must include not only a complete description of the survey results but also an account of the survey instrument itself, including the design and development process, validation efforts, and how the survey was administered. The benefits of comprehensive survey reporting are summarized in Box 4.

Table 16 lists several sets of survey reporting guidelines available in the literature, and a full recommended checklist of reporting guidelines based on the work of Artino et al.[2] is included at the end of this chapter. Although general conventions for organizing survey findings may be inferred from reading survey studies published in reputable health professions education (HPE) journals, not all published articles represent best practices according to the guidelines in Table 16.[3,4] This chapter fleshes out some of these guidelines, focusing on the practical issues that especially challenge survey designers (researchers and educators) when they are reporting survey studies. The recommendations presented are based on the literature and on the authors' salient experiences as scholars, reviewers, and journal editors. Not every point on the checklist that concludes this chapter is covered in the text that follows.

> **BOX 4 ■ The Benefits of Comprehensive Survey Reporting**
>
> Comprehensive survey reporting...
> - Allows readers to assess the degree to which the survey yielded credible data from which valid inferences can be made;
> - Helps readers judge the potential relevance of the survey instrument for use in their own contexts;
> - Gives reviewers and editors the information needed to evaluate if the survey study is trustworthy and fit for publication; and
> - Facilitates survey reuse, study replication, and knowledge syntheses (e.g., systematic reviews and meta-analyses).

TABLE 16 ■ A List of Survey Reporting Guidelines From the Literature

Checklist	Notes	Source	QR Code
Bennett et al.[6]	Combination of Kelly et al., Burns et al., Draugalis et al., and AAPOR. The most comprehensive checklist.	https://bit.ly/2kxEA1x	
Kelley et al.[7]	Author subjective recommendations. Focuses on paradata.	https://bit.ly/2zgOqa4	
Burns et al.[8]	Author subjective recommendations but not in checklist format.	https://bit.ly/38jZaGc	
Draugalis et al.[9]	Authors' modified version of AAPOR checklist. Focuses on validity and reliability.	https://bit.ly/39kWFUn	
AAPOR[10]	Broad guidelines without granular checklist.	https://bit.ly/2QbKzTW	
Eysenbach[11]	Author subjective opinion, Internet-specific.	https://bit.ly/2m4u1n5	
Artino et al.[2]	Serves as *Academic Medicine's* survey reporting guidelines.	https://bit.ly/3aZqOKE	

Note: A multitude of guidelines for various study methods can be found on the EQUATOR Network's website (https://www.equator-network.org/reporting-guidelines/).

The remainder of this chapter is organized by the sections found in the typical original research article: "Introduction," "Methods," "Results," and "Discussion." It is important to note, however, that there are very few "always" rules for how or where survey information should be reported. These suggestions offer a starting point for what must be a conscientious and reflective writing process. In their *Academic Medicine* "Last Page" article, Lingard and Watling[5] argued that good research articles emphasize the "Methods" and "Results," but great research articles incorporate what was done and what happened into an engaging and persuasive story. This larger narrative, which unfolds in the "Introduction" and "Discussion" gives effective research articles a clear setting, purpose, and audience; and the narrative guides implications for future study. From this perspective, quality survey reporting includes demonstrating how the survey and its results advance the pursuit of the study objectives and research questions.

 VOICE OF EXPERIENCE

Although manuscripts typically have standard locations for where to put certain information, authors are encouraged to position reporting information in the location that best suits the story being told in a given study. A good example of this is reliability and validity evidence, which can fit in either the "Methods" or "Results" (or both), depending on the study purpose and the manuscript's intended audience. The most important point is that the necessary information is provided and contributes meaningfully to the overall story of the research.

Technically, most survey studies are prospective observational studies, but the STROBE guidelines, which are designed for observational studies, are not entirely relevant. In addition, there is no single accepted set of guidelines for surveys. Ultimately, there is no right or wrong set of guidelines to use. Nonetheless, the important point is to use a published checklist and cite it in the manuscript, just as with any other reporting guidelines.

A survey-based research manuscript, therefore, should include the necessary information identified by reporting guidelines in a way that flows well and tells the best story of the work performed. So, in addition to asking, "What and how much information should be reported?" it is also important to ask, "What do the data gathered have to say about the issue investigated? What information is essential to convey that message to the intended audience?" Using a patient case analogy, questions might be: "What are the pertinent findings that support the diagnosis? How should the physician present these findings to a colleague who is interested in this case?"

Introduction

PROVIDE A RATIONALE FOR USING A SURVEY

Helpful general guidance for writing effective introductions is readily available in the literature.[5,12] This guidance highlights the importance of clearly identifying the conceptual or practical problem being addressed and making a strong argument for why the chosen research design effectively accomplishes this task. When reporting a survey study, this means clearly articulating why a survey instrument was the best tool for the job. Surveys are ideal for measuring things that are not directly observable, including attitudes, opinions, and beliefs, such as residents' satisfaction with feedback or medical students' experiences in a classroom. However, lack of direct visibility of respondents' behavior can come at the cost of meaningfulness. For example, a course evaluation survey can easily measure learner satisfaction, but it likely cannot assess students' actual learning or behavior changes. Survey designers must articulate clearly how they managed such limitations and why it made sense to use a survey to answer their research questions.

A common location to describe the rationale is in the "Introduction" section or near the top of the "Methods" section, where the study design is described (see Box 5).[13] If using multiple methods, such as a survey plus exam scores or semistructured interviews, it is important to explain the connection between the methods, specifically, how the different sources of data are intended to answer the research questions in an integrated and comprehensive fashion.

BOX 5 ■ Example of Survey Rationale Statement[13]

"To measure the frequency of serious research misconduct and other questionable research practices (QRPs), many different approaches have been employed. These include counts of confirmed cases of researcher fraud and paper retractions, as well as research audits by government funders. Such methods are limited because they are calculated based on misconduct that has been discovered, and detecting such misconduct is difficult. Moreover, distinguishing intentional misconduct from honest mistakes is challenging. Therefore such approaches significantly underestimate the real frequency of misconduct and QRPs, because only researchers know if they have willfully acted in an unethical or questionable manner.

To address these challenges, survey methods have been used to directly ask scientists about their research behaviors. Like the measurement of any socially undesirable behavior, assessing irresponsible research practices via self-report likely underestimates the true prevalence or frequency of the behaviors. Nonetheless, when employed appropriately, survey methods can generate reasonable estimates that provide a general sense of the problem's scope."

Methods

DESCRIBE HOW THE SURVEY INSTRUMENT WAS CREATED OR ADAPTED FROM EXISTING SURVEY(S)

Survey designers should provide a complete and thorough description of how their survey was created or how it was adapted from a previously published survey instrument. Similarly, an explanation for *not* using a previously published instrument, if available, is important. Information that is typically provided includes: (1) how prior survey tools were searched for and found (or not found); (2) the qualifications of the item writers; and (3) the sequence of creation, from construct conception to survey drafts to pretesting and pilot testing. If a previously published survey was translated from another language, the process used to conduct the translation and verify its accuracy should be reported in the "Methods" section as well. A separate subsection in the "Methods," such as "Instrument Development," can help readers locate this type of information.

DISCUSS HOW THE SURVEY INSTRUMENT WAS PRETESTED PRIOR TO FULL IMPLEMENTATION

A critical part of describing how the instrument was made is describing the pretesting activities. Every survey tool, especially new or adapted surveys, should be pretested and the process detailed in the manuscript. Pretesting (described in **Step 2: Survey Construction** and **Step 3: Establishing Evidence**) includes activities like expert reviews, cognitive interviewing, and pilot testing, all of which can help establish evidence that the content of the survey is complete and that respondents understand (and can answer) the questions being asked. The level of detail in explaining the pretesting activities should be enough to allow others to fully understand what was done and thus replicate the study if desired. Examples of information to provide are: (1) the number of experts, their qualifications, and whether all stakeholders were represented; (2) the number and background of the people who provided the cognitive interviews and completed the pilot test; (3) the degree to which those who completed the pilot test accurately represent the larger study sample; and, in some cases, (4) a summary of the changes made to the survey as a result of the pretesting activities (see Box 6).[14]

PROVIDE THE FINAL SURVEY INSTRUMENT

Survey designers should provide a complete, formatted copy of the survey instrument for inclusion in the article's appendix or online-only supplemental materials (more on these later). An exported PDF or word processing document is ideal because it allows readers to see exactly what respondents saw when they took the survey.

BOX 6 ■ Example of Reporting Pretesting Activities[14]

"A 16-item survey consisting of Likert-type and narrative response items was created. Cognitive pre-testing, specifically a think-aloud approach, was used to ensure correct understanding of the questions. After minor revisions, the updated survey version retested successfully. The instrument was then pre-tested by 11 individuals representing all specialties in the sampling frame. No concerns were raised, and initial data from the 11 individuals approximated what we expected."

VOICE OF EXPERIENCE

Simply providing an abridged version of each survey item in a table or figure is insufficient instrument reporting, as is copy/pasting the item stems without also including the labeled response options. These practices are insufficient because wording and formatting can make a significant difference (statistically and practically) in survey responses. The most transparent and recommended way to describe the instrument is to share the actual instrument or an exported version of an online instrument with readers.

DETAIL HOW AND WHEN THE SURVEY INSTRUMENT WAS ADMINISTERED

Survey-based research articles must include not only the final version of the survey but also a description of how the survey was administered. Key decisions made as part of **Step 4: Survey Delivery** should be included, from incentives and prenotifications to who delivered the instrument, when the survey took place, and the timing of invitations and reminders. Sometimes relative timing is more important to report than exact dates. For example, consider two identical surveys about academic stress: one administered shortly before and one shortly after residency match. These may produce widely divergent results (and have widely divergent response rates) resulting from the effects of stress and anxiety on survey respondents themselves. Also important is the survey format (Web-based, paper-based, or interview formats), whether or not the survey was anonymous, and how much time was given to complete it.

Manuscript length limitations require thoughtful decisions about which details to present in the "Methods" section versus an appendix or online-only supplement. When making these decisions, it is important to understand how survey implementation shapes not only who responds but also how they process the survey items. Readers of survey-based reports should be able to judge whether and how the implementation approach influenced the meaning of the data gathered. Also, research surveys are often usable beyond the study for which they were designed, and information about implementation context is critically important if readers are to evaluate how far survey instruments can faithfully transfer to other contexts with or without modification.

Results

DESCRIBE THE SURVEY RESPONDENTS, RESPONSE RATE, AND HOW NONRESPONSE BIAS WAS ASSESSED

Before going on to more detailed findings designed to answer their research questions, survey designers should first give readers a sense of what happened when they administered the survey. Specifically, designers should report who completed the survey and how completely they responded to the items. As already noted, this kind of information is a key part of clarifying the limitations of the findings and understanding what might happen with a different sample under different conditions.

BOX 7 ■ Example of Respondent Reporting[15]

"From the initial sample of 391 email addresses, 54 email contacts were returned as undeliverable, yielding 337 valid email addresses. According to the Qualtrics platform, 141 respondents opened the survey and 109 completed it, representing an overall response rate of 32.3% (109/337). A comparison of the characteristics of initial versus postreminder survey respondents found no significant differences in gender, academic rank, highest degree, area of study highest degree, region, years of experience in medical education, or peer-reviewed publications in the past two years."

Respondents

Generally speaking, reporting about study participants should characterize the people who completed the survey (i.e., sample size, basic demographic characteristics; see Box 7).[15] When a survey is cross-sectional or given at multiple institutions, participant information specific to each cohort or institution is often provided, unless providing such information is incompatible with the study design (e.g., medical schools in a multiinstitutional study of well-being may decide they want to present only aggregated results). And when a survey is given on multiple occasions longitudinally, participant information should be provided for each administration and attrition noted.

Response Rate

The response rate should be reported using one of the six official American Association for Public Opinion Research (AAPOR)[16] response rate definitions discussed in **Step 5: Data Analysis**, if possible. If none of those definitions are appropriate for a study, then a detailed custom definition should be reported. For example, a statement like "The final total number of responses was 371, yielding a response rate of 67%, AAPOR Definition 2," concisely conveys the total number of potential respondents, actual number of respondents, whether authors were confident of potential respondent eligibility, and whether partial responses were included in the results, all of which are essential for readers to interpret the findings properly.

Nonresponse Bias

There is no "magic number" below which nonresponse bias becomes a problem (and, for that matter, above which it is *not* a problem). It is possible to have a 20% response rate but not have nonresponse bias. Similarly, it is possible to have an 80% response rate and still have nonresponse bias.[17] The key is transparency: survey designers should report how they assessed nonresponse bias and, where applicable, whether anything was done to correct for it (e.g., using a stratified sample or analyzing respondent patterns over time). Adjusting for nonresponse bias is like addressing confounders in regressions, so it may be reasonable to report both raw and adjusted data. Readers are encouraged to review **Step 5: Data Analysis** and look elsewhere[17,18] for more thorough discussions of nonresponse bias and ways to correct for it.

PROVIDE EVIDENCE OF RELIABILITY AND VALIDITY

The framework used to collect and report reliability and validity evidence is often introduced in the "Methods" section, and reliability and validity data are typically presented in the "Results" section, especially when the study is an instrument development and validation study. However, such reliability and validity evidence can also be presented in the "Methods" section. Furthermore, the rationale for the choice of validity framework is important to share, usually in the "Methods" section, because how validity (and reliability) evidence is presented depends on that framework (see **Step 3: Establishing Evidence** for framework details).

> **BOX 8 ■ Example of Validity Framework[19]**
>
> "We used DeVellis's 8-step framework to develop the tool, and Messick's unified theory of validity informed our validation approach. In addition, our approach to validation was informed by van der Vleuten's utility formula for consideration for the tool acceptability."

VOICE OF EXPERIENCE

The answer to the question, "Where do we report our validation efforts?" often varies according to the study purpose and design and journal preferences. As discussed in **Step 3: Establishing Evidence**, a helpful guiding principle is: If the validation was background to the main purpose of the study (e.g., the main purpose is to showcase the survey results, which help answer a substantive research question), then validity evidence results probably fit best in the "Methods" section. On the other hand, if validation is the main purpose of the study (e.g., developing and testing a new survey instrument), then validity evidence results might be best reported in the "Results" section.

Typically, the presentation is one to two paragraphs describing each of the sources of validity in turn, with evidence to support them (see Box 8).[19] There is often a blur between the "Methods" and "Results" sections because some sources, such as content validity (e.g., expert reviews), might be reported in the "Methods" section, whereas something like "relationships with other variables" may be reported in the "Results" section as part of study findings for the primary and secondary objectives (e.g., correlation between survey items or scales and other variables measured in the study).

Finally, survey designers should report reliability and validity statistics for each survey instrument (or survey scale) used in the study, based on data *from their sample*. Reporting reliability and validity statistics from prior studies that used the survey (with a different sample) may be appropriate for establishing the survey's credibility and supporting the proposed use of the tool, but doing so should not substitute for also reporting reliability and validity statistics for the survey responses in the current study.

PRESENT RESULTS AND ANALYSES IN A CONCISE AND EASILY INTERPRETABLE FORMAT

Similar to novice physicians' case reports, novice survey designers' reports of survey findings can be overly comprehensive and obscure the key points, or they can be overly simplified and exclude important details, thereby introducing error in interpretation and use. Common questions about how to report survey findings include: "What information should be reported? How much information is too much (or too little)? How should the information be grouped?" For better or worse, these questions do not have one right answer. It depends on the story being told and the audience to which it is being told, as mentioned at the beginning of this chapter.

VOICE OF EXPERIENCE

Some survey designers make a separate internal document with all of the data—far more than should be reported—and make an outline of the "Results" section from that internal document first (much like an outline of a manuscript) to easily move information around to best narrate the findings. For example, should all of the study's data be presented sequentially—i.e., items to scales to inferential findings? Or should the item information and inferential findings be reported separately for each scale used? The answer is whatever will logically tell the most informative story. But the key point is that survey designers can use a data outline to try out different narratives to see which works best.

Item Data

Basic quantitative item data include means (or medians), standard deviations (or modes), frequency counts, and percentages for each item in the survey. These data can convey important information about how the survey respondents approached completing the survey, and they may reveal influences on participant responses that are not those that the survey designer sought to study. For example, items with very high or low means and very small standard deviations may suggest that respondents felt pressure (directly or indirectly) to respond in a particular way. This is not an uncommon phenomenon when people are asked to report on their own or others' socially desirable (or undesirable) attitudes or behaviors,[20] and it can negatively affect the validity of the survey scores (see **Step 3: Establishing Evidence**). Another important reason for reporting quantitative item data is to justify the selection of statistical tests (such as parametric or nonparametric analyses).

The decision of whether to present items in tables with means and standard deviations, tables with medians and modes, tables with ranked anchors, histograms, or just written text depends on how the data are best interpreted (see **Step 5: Data Analysis** for categorical versus ratio and interval arguments). Analysis requirements can also dictate how data are presented. For example, if assumptions of normality are violated by the data distribution, then the data should probably be analyzed with nonparametric tests, for which medians and modes with histograms are more appropriate than means and standard deviations. Presenting every single item in histogram form, though, can quickly become bulky, and tables are difficult to create and interpret if the response options are not the same. A histogram is *not* encouraged for every item and rarely is helpful for even a single item, an exception being an important stratification comparison that is explicitly linked to a research question.

If the data are reasonably interpreted as continuous, means with standard deviations for each item can simply be written in the text for each item (or for each scale score; see Box 9[21] and later in this chapter). Readers can be referred to the instrument (another reason that providing the full and final instrument is so important) for the full set of response options, or they can be described in the text with the means. It is important to include the response options, though, to provide context for numbers. For example, "Students were generally satisfied with the course, 4.2 ± 0.5," is meaningless without the context of the response options, where 1 = *Not at all satisfied* and 5 = *Extremely satisfied*. Referring readers to the full instrument for every item is also not ideal because it distracts from the story being developed.

If the data are best interpreted as categorical, the frequency percentages for each response option are often reported. The total or actual number of responses should be reported with percentages so that readers can back-calculate the raw frequencies (see Box 10).[22] In addition, if an instrument employed several items with categorical response options, they can be easily compiled into a table. If the data do not fit well in a table, authors might consider presenting such data visually, using histograms, stacked bar charts (see Fig. 6), or other graphical visualizations.

It is not always necessary to report the item-level results of a survey in the "Results" section. For example, if the study objectives are evaluating variables around a scale, such as the Maslach Burnout Inventory,[23] it is the scale scores that are important, not the individual item scores within the scale (see additional information on scales later in this chapter). In the spirit of data transparency,

---

BOX 9 ■ Example of Continuous Data Reported in Text[21]

"The range of values for the summative pimping score was 13 to 42 (potential range of 11–50), with a mean and median of 24 and a normal distribution (Shapiro-Wilk p = .4). The quartile cutoffs for this score were: first quartile ≤ 20 (n = 32), second quartile 21–23 (n = 30), third quartile 24–27 (n = 33), and fourth quartile ≥ 28 (n = 30)."

BOX 10 ■ Example of Categorical Data Reported in Text[22]

"The majority of students used their personal phones to communicate with medical team members about patient-related matters (86%, 85/99) and nonpatient-related matters (93%, 92/99). Although 71% (70/99) of students had password protection on their phones, the survey revealed that 26% (26/99) of students' phones lacked any type of security feature."

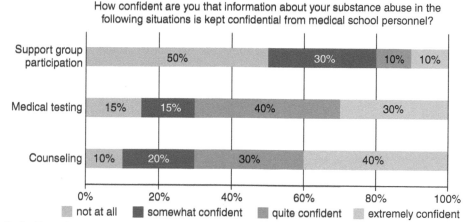

How confident are you that information about your substance abuse in the following situations is kept confidential from medical school personnel?

Fig. 6 Example of a horizontal stacked bar chart for presenting categorical data using the **Book Introduction** example case.

it may be advisable to include item-level responses somewhere, such as in an appendix, but apart from validity and reliability analyses, the item scores do not have as much meaning as the overall scale or subscale scores.

Scale Data

As discussed in **Step 2: Survey Construction**, survey scales are often used to measure more complex constructs. For example, the Motivated Strategies for Learning Questionnaire[24] attempts to capture several course-specific aspects of motivation and self-regulated learning and includes several subscales intended to measure motivational components (e.g., self-efficacy, task value, and test anxiety) and regulatory strategies (e.g., critical thinking and effort regulation).

Presenting scale or subscale data gives the reader a sense for how well they represent their respective constructs and, by extension, how much confidence the reader should have in the additional analyses done with those scale scores or the conclusions drawn about the constructs they were intended to measure. Scales may function more or less well as construct operationalizations, depending on sample and context; this is why scale data are important to report in each study where a scale is used, especially if use deviates from the intentions of the scale's creators. Scale data to report include scale means and standard deviations and internal consistency reliability estimates (often reported as Cronbach's alpha; see Table 17).[25] In more detailed and sophisticated survey instrument validation efforts, survey designers may also choose to report the intercorrelations of items on a scale or subscale in addition to the results of dimensional analyses, such as exploratory or confirmatory factor analysis, generalizability studies, or Rasch modeling. Detailing how to report the findings of these more advanced analyses is beyond the scope of this book, but several helpful resources exist to assist.[26–28]

TABLE 17 ■ Descriptive Statistics, Cronbach's Alpha and Pearson's Correlations for the Study[25]

Variable	Mean	SD	Items, n	α	1	2	3	4	5	6	7
1 Task value	4.45	0.48	6	0.85	-	0.39†	0.51†	-0.08	-0.28‡	0.26‡	0.01
2 Self-efficacy	3.77	0.70	4	0.85		-	0.27‡	-0.36†	-0.23†	0.17	0.08
3 Enjoyment	3.76	0.56	4	0.76			-	-0.24‡	-0.30†	0.16	0.2†
4 Anxiety	3.01	0.80	4	0.81				-	0.03	-0.25‡	-0.19†
5 Boredom	2.69	0.84	3	0.81						-0.26‡	-0.16
6 Course exam grade	82.62	5.86	-	-						-	0.64†
7 NBME shelf exam score	547.35	86.92	-	-							-

†$p < 0.001$; ‡$p < 0.01$, T$p < 0.05$. All subscale variables were measured on a 5-point agreement response scale. NBME National Board of Medical Examiners; SD, standard deviation.

Inferential Data

Often, survey studies explore the interrelations among multiple constructs, such as the associations between empathy, spirituality, and burnout. Depending on the research questions being addressed, the relationships among demographic variables, survey items, and/or survey scales might be of interest as well. Although descriptive data are traditionally reported first, followed by inferential statistics, the "Results" narrative can sometimes best be portrayed by reporting inferential statistics with descriptive data.

Combining Quantitative and Qualitative Data

When surveys capture quantitative (numerical) and qualitative (open-ended, free text) data, figuring out where to put the qualitative results can be challenging. Should the qualitative results come after the quantitative? Alternatively, should the results be presented in the order in which the survey items were administered? If there is more than one open-ended item, should the qualitative results for all items be presented together? The short, yet unsatisfying, answer to these questions is: "It depends." It depends on what the open-ended items asked of respondents and how the answers to these items relate to making sense of the survey's quantitative items. Qualitative findings should be placed where they naturally occur in the story being told, aiding readers' understanding of the theoretical and/or practical phenomena being investigated.

Generally, there are two main ways qualitative data are presented in survey studies: (1) in conjunction with a quantitative item as the "Other" option, and (2) as stand-alone, written response items (i.e., open-ended by design). Often the open-ended responses to "Other" will be infrequent and sparse, and if they make up an inconsequential percentage of the responses (at the authors' and editors' discretion), it is often reasonable to report the most commonly occurring responses in the text. However, if "Other" responses constitute a practically meaningful proportion, such as 5% to 10%, it may be appropriate for the open-ended responses to undergo some type of replicable, documented, content analysis and then be reported in the text (or in an appendix) with frequencies and example quotations. Note that interpreting such responses should be done with caution because high rates of "Other" responses implies that the response options given were insufficient, and thus many respondents responded differently than expected. Sometimes, in such circumstances, items must be removed from the formal analysis. Either way, full disclosure of the decisions made should be reported in the manuscript.

When survey items are open-ended by design, it may be appropriate to analyze responses using a more systematic qualitative approach, such as thematic analysis (see **Step 5: Data Analysis**). Ideally, open-ended items on a survey are designed to gather data that are not readily quantified or that offer more depth than what is captured by the quantitative items. For instance, a common use of open-ended items in education surveys is to gather slightly more detailed information about why respondents thought a particular course was useful and what they would recommend to improve it. These items typically accompany quantitative items assessing respondent satisfaction with the course and instructor. To tell the relatively straightforward story of respondents' perceptions of the course, it may be simplest to present the qualitative results altogether, just after the quantitative data. This approach would allow readers to first gauge overall level of satisfaction and then explore the possible factors influencing those satisfaction ratings.

However, important caveats for applying qualitative methods to survey data exist, and many times including open-ended survey questions is a poor choice for survey designers trying to capture the kind of rich, descriptive data necessary for credible qualitative analysis.[29] Careful consideration should be given to whether research questions characteristic of high-quality qualitative approaches should be addressed using self-report survey items[30]; in many cases, the answer to this question is an emphatic, "No."

Combining Tables, Figures, and Text

The old adage, "A picture is worth a thousand words," is particularly true when reporting survey findings, especially in HPE journals, which often have fairly restrictive word limits. The key objective is to strike the right balance among text, tables, and figures. After all, most journals have limitations on tables and figures, too. More importantly, using text, tables, and figures according to their purpose helps tell the story in a concise yet engaging and meaningful way.

The best role for tables and figures in survey studies is usually to express comparisons, and thus any associated text should usually be used to highlight important points. If authors find themselves discussing every item in a table, then the table is probably unnecessary.[31] It is worth repeating that graphs, histograms, and tables for individual items are discouraged because they require excessive real estate and provide no more information than words in the text.

Blocks of Likert-type items (i.e., those using the same response options) can also be presented in tables, and comparisons provided in distal columns as applicable. The presentation order of the items in the table can be different from the order in the instrument if that helps visually present comparisons and if the actual instrument is provided with the manuscript.

Sometimes an instrument is especially large or includes several scales, and thus it is not feasible or meaningful to include the frequencies for every option of every response option in the body of the manuscript. One way to nonetheless provide the full results is to include the frequencies and percentages adjacent to each item in the copy of the survey instrument provided to readers, which is usually included in an appendix.

 VOICE OF EXPERIENCE

Different journals have different expectations for formatting text, tables, and figures. The recommendations provided here should be applied along with careful review of the instructions to authors provided by the journal where the manuscript is being submitted. In general, it is good practice to develop a thorough understanding of what specific editors want by inspecting the journals' author instructions, previously published papers, and guidance detailed in their editorials, to present the research in the best light possible.

Discussion

DISCUSS FINDINGS IN RELATION TO STUDY OBJECTIVES AND RESEARCH QUESTIONS, AND DESCRIBE STUDY LIMITATIONS AND GENERALIZABILITY

Once the results have been reported, the story comes to completion in the "Discussion" section. The "Results" section, which is carefully organized to highlight the findings that speak directly to the research questions and the overarching study objectives, should lead readers easily to this point. The "Discussion" section often begins by summarizing the key findings in relation to the hypotheses (if applicable) and then goes on to evaluate for readers the ways in which the results advance (or not) the study narrative. In addition, the "Discussion" section should honestly outline the limitations of the study and the degree to which the findings might generalize or transfer to other contexts (e.g., different settings, persons, and outcomes).

For many survey designers, writing the "Discussion" is challenging for at least two reasons. First, the "Discussion" section tends to be less formulaic than, for example, the "Methods" and "Results" sections. As such, the "Discussion" can sometimes require a bit more creativity on the part of authors. Second, by this point in the writing process, the other sections of the paper have already been drafted and the survey designers may be somewhat weary. Although it is beyond the scope of this chapter to discuss all the nuances of how to write a good "Discussion" section, interested readers are encouraged to review guidance provided elsewhere.[32]

> ### BOX 11 ■ Recommended Paradata: Minimum Checklist
>
> - Details of respondent eligibility
> - How the response rate was calculated
> - Details of survey creation, pretesting, and validation (e.g., credentials of expert reviewers, cognitive interviewing details)
> - Details of survey administration (e.g., call logs, characteristics of interviewers)
>
> ---
>
> *Note:* Specifics will vary by the methods and instrument(s) used. No formal recommendations exist for a minimum standard.[35]

VOICE OF EXPERIENCE

Alignment between the "Introduction" and "Discussion" may be improved by outlining both sections in side-by-side format. This technique helps to visualize how and where the "Discussion" section revisits the questions raised in the "Introduction" section, builds on the gaps identified, and points toward future research and practice. It can also reveal where the "Discussion" section strays beyond the data and needs refinement to keep the story grounded.

Appendices

Appendices are useful tools for meeting the reporting guidelines featured in this chapter in addition to meeting journal word limitations. Appendices are sometimes included as a component of the published article but more often show up as supplemental "Online only" material. Deciding what to put in an appendix involves determining which information is essential to telling the story and interpreting the study (and thus should go in the main body of the manuscript) versus which material is useful for taking a "deeper dive" for purposes other than understanding the main story (e.g., the potential efficacy of the survey in a different target population in a different setting). A good example of supplemental information is the complete survey instrument, which should be discussed in the text but is often best presented, in full, in an appendix for space reasons.

Appendices included in published articles can also provide detailed information that is helpful to interpret the findings but could occlude the main message if presented in the article's body because it is not essential information. Examples include factor loadings from factor structure techniques, alternative structural equation models tested, subgroup findings (e.g., differential patterns of responding by people of differing gender, race/ethnicity, year of study, academic performance, etc.), or components of the survey that were used as part of a larger study.

Some of the other information requested in survey reporting checklists falls under the category of paradata, and much of it is often appropriate for an appendix. The term "paradata" refers to administrative data about the survey and the processes used to collect the data. As such, paradata can help readers better understand the context of survey administration and, if desired, can help them replicate the study. Deciding which paradata to report is really up to the authors, and these decisions will vary by survey topic, objectives, sampling frame, delivery mode, and other factors. Nonetheless, Box 11 lists paradata that are often reported in appendixes. The U.S. Centers for Disease Control and Prevention (CDC) does an excellent job of providing paradata for its surveys, and a good example is the National Health Interview Survey, although this represents the highest degree of presentation and disclosure, which is not necessary for most surveys.[33]

Another best practice that aligns with open science recommendations is to share survey data and paradata on free data-sharing repositories such as Figshare (https://figshare.com). Data sharing has many potential benefits, including but not limited to greater transparency and collaboration, increased confidence in findings, and enhanced goodwill among investigators.[34]

Chapter Summary

This chapter provides guidelines for what reviewers, editors, and other discerning readers look for in research reports that include surveys. However, sometimes mitigating circumstances may limit the development and reporting of a survey. For instance, surveys of disaster victims may need to prioritize timeliness over other aspects of survey development. In such cases there may not be time to pretest questions in the way that could occur when time is not so critical. There also are limitations in funding to carry out many of the elements of survey design, and these limitations may be difficult to overcome, particularly for surveys developed by trainees. A creative, innovative idea embedded in a survey that has design limitations may still offer important insights. As long as those limitations can be clearly identified, and the results of the survey can be understood in the context of those boundaries, there may be value in sharing the information with the academic community in a peer-reviewed article.

Surveys provide important information that can guide our understanding of educational innovations and current challenges facing the academic community. The purpose of this chapter is to encourage thoughtful and complete reporting of survey-based research in addition to other survey design and development efforts. Investigators are encouraged to use surveys to ask important questions and to share their findings with the HPE community. By following this and other relevant guidance,[1,28,36–38] the time spent on survey projects will be more productive and valuable to the scientific community. What is more, by following these reporting guidelines, survey-based research articles will have better odds of being published in the peer-reviewed literature and used again (or adapted) by other scholars. In the end, the outcome of better surveys and survey reporting will be better educational research and evaluation.

*Portions of this chapter were previously published in *Academic Medicine* and are used with express permission of the publisher, Wolters Kluwer.[2]

Reporting Guidelines Checklist

Reporting guideline	*Questions to address in the manuscript*
Introduction	
Provide a rationale for using a survey method.[a]	☐ Why is a survey an appropriate data collection method? ☐ How can the research question(s) be answered using a survey?
Methods	
Describe how the survey instrument was created or adapted from existing survey(s).	☐ How were the survey items developed? ☐ What literature was reviewed? ☐ How do the survey items relate to the construct of interest? ☐ If applicable, what changes were made to previously published surveys and why?

Discuss how the survey instrument was pretested prior to full implementation.	☐ Were experts used to pretest the survey?
	    ☐ If so, describe their qualifications, how many experts were consulted, and what the review process was like.
	☐ Were cognitive interviews conducted?
	    ☐ If so, describe the interviewees, how many were interviewed, and what the interviewing procedures were like.
	☐ Was a pilot test conducted?
	    ☐ If so, describe the sample size, the types of participants, and how the pilot test was conducted.

Provide the final survey instrument.	☐ Has a complete, formatted copy of the survey been included in the article or appendix?
Detail how and when the survey instrument was administered.	☐ Has the content of the final survey draft been described in detail (e.g., number and types of items and response options)? ☐ What was the method of survey administration (e.g., Web-based, paper-based, interview), and where and when was the survey administered? ☐ Was the survey anonymous or otherwise confidential? ☐ How were respondents contacted and how often? ☐ How long did respondents have to complete the survey? ☐ Were respondents compensated for completing the survey?
Results	
Describe the survey respondents, response rate, and how nonresponse bias was assessed	☐ Who comprises the sample and how does the sample relate to the population of interest? ☐ What was the response rate, and how was it calculated? ☐ Was nonresponse bias assessed and, if so, what was done to account for it?

(Continued)

Reporting guideline	Questions to address in the manuscript
Provide evidence of reliability and validity.[b]	☐ What processes and statistics were used to assess the reliability of the survey scores? ☐ What sources of validity evidence were collected and how do they support the intended use of the survey results? 　☐ At a minimum, content and response process validity should be considered (e.g., through expert reviews and cognitive interviewing). 　☐ Avoid using so-called "face validity" as evidence, because most measurement experts agree that it is not a legitimate source of validity evidence.[39] ☐ If applicable, which type of validity framework was used to guide survey development and validation? For example, Messick's[40] five sources of validity evidence or Kane's[41] framework. ☐ See **Step 3: Establishing Evidence** for more details on frameworks and processes for collecting reliability and validity evidence.
Present results and analyses in a concise and easily interpretable format.	☐ Have only the most important results been reported in the main body of the manuscript? 　☐ Present the data in a logical way that clearly conveys the most important findings. ☐ Are the tables and figures clearly labeled, necessary, and not overly redundant with the text? ☐ Are the numbers in the tables, figures, and text consistent?

Discussion

Discuss findings in relation to study objectives and research questions and describe study limitations and generalizability.	☐ How do findings relate to the study objectives and research questions? 　☐ Appropriately interpret findings in light of study limitations. 　☐ Consider alternative interpretations and refute those that are not credible. ☐ What caveats should be considered when interpreting the results? ☐ What are the implications for research and practice? ☐ What conclusions can be drawn? 　☐ Novice and expert survey designers alike often draw inappropriate conclusions from limited survey results. This practice should be avoided. 　☐ When in doubt, make conservative inferences, claims, and conclusions that are supported by the survey method used and the data collected. ☐ What are the limitations (and strengths) of using a survey to address the research questions? ☐ To what extent can the findings be generalized to other contexts (e.g., different settings, persons, and outcomes)?

[a]The rationale can also be presented in the "Methods" section.
[b]Reliability and validity evidence are often presented elsewhere in a survey research report (e.g., "Introduction," "Methods," or even "Discussion" sections).

References

1. Dillman DA, Smyth JD, Christian LM. *Internet, Phone, Mail, and Mixed-Mode Surveys: The Tailored Design Method.* 4th ed. Hoboken, NJ: John Wiley & Sons, Inc; 2014.
2. Artino AR, Durning SJ, Sklar DP. Guidelines for reporting survey-based research submitted to Academic Medicine. *Acad Med.* 2018;93(3):337–340. doi:10.1097/ACM. 0000000000002094.
3. Artino AR, Phillips AW, Utrankar A, Ta AQ, Durning SJ. The questions shape the answers: assessing the quality of published survey instruments in health professions education. *Acad Med.* 2018;93(3):456–463.
4. Phillips AW, Friedman BT, Utrankar A, Ta AQ, Reddy ST, Durning SJ. Surveys of health professions trainees: prevalence, response rates, and predictive factors to guide researchers. *Acad Med.* 2017;92(2):222–228.
5. Lingard L, Watling C. It's a story. Not a study. *Acad Med.* 2016;91(12):e12. doi:10.1097/ACM. 0000000000001389.
6. Bennett C, Khangura S, Brehaut JC, et al. Reporting guidelines for survey research: an analysis of published guidance and reporting practices. *PLoS Med.* 2011; 8(8):e1001069. doi:10.1371/journal. pmed.1001069.
7. Kelley K. Good practice in the conduct and reporting of survey research. *Int J Qual Heal Care.* 2003;15(3):261–266. doi:10.1093/intqhc/mzg031.
8. Burns KEA, Duffett M, Kho ME, et al. A guide for the design and conduct of self-administered surveys of clinicians. *CMAJ.* 2008;179(3):245–252. doi:10.1503/cmaj.080372.
9. Draugalis JR, Coons SJ, Plaza CM. Best practices for survey research reports: a synopsis for authors and reviewers. *Am J Pharm Educ.* 2008;72(1):11. doi:10.5688/aj720111.
10. Best Practices for Survey Research—AAPOR. https://www.aapor.org/Standards-Ethics/Best-Practices. aspx. Accessed February 11, 2020.
11. Eysenbach G. Improving the quality of Web surveys: the Checklist for Reporting Results of Internet E-Surveys (CHERRIES). *J Med Internet Res.* 2004;6(3):e34. doi:10.2196/jmir.6.3.e34.
12. Lingard L. Joining a conversation: the problem/gap/hook heuristic. *Perspect Med Educ.* 2015;4(5):252–253. doi:10.1007/s40037-015-0211-y.
13. Artino AR, Driessen EW, Maggio LA. Ethical Shades of Gray: International Frequency of Scientific Misconduct and Questionable Research Practices in Health Professions Education, Academic Medicine. 2019;94(1):76–84. doi: 10.1097/ACM.0000000000002412.
14. Yin I, Phillips A, Straus CM. Best reporting practices for multipart CT scans: A pilot evaluation and construction of the optimal analysis methodology. *J Am Coll Radiol.* 2019;16(10):1409–1415. doi:10.1016/j. jacr.2019.02.046.
15. Uijtdehaage S, Mavis B, Durning SJ. Whose paper is it anyway? Authorship criteria according to established scholars in health professions education. *Acad Med.* ePub ahead of print.
16. The American Association for Public Opinion Research. *Standard Definitions: Final Dispositions of Case Codes and Outcome Rates for Surveys.* 9th ed. AAPOR; 2016.
17. Groves RM, Peytcheva E. The impact of nonresponse rates on nonresponse bias: a meta-analysis. *Public Opin Q.* 2008;72(2):167–189. doi:10.1093/poq/nfn011.
18. Phillips AW, Reddy S, Durning SJ. Improving response rates and evaluating nonresponse bias in surveys: AMEE Guide No. 102. *Med Teach.* 2016;38(3):217–228. doi:10.3109/0142159X. 2015.1105945.
19. St-Onge C, Young M, Varpio L. Development and validation of a health profession education-focused scholarly mentorship assessment tool. *Perspect Med Educ.* 2019;8(1):43–46. doi:10.1007/s40037-018-0491-0.
20. Dudek NL, Marks MB, Regehr G. Failure to fail: the perspectives of clinical supervisors. *Acad Med.* 2005;80(10 Suppl):S84–S87.
21. McEvoy JW, Shatzer JH, Desai SV, Wright SM. Questioning style and pimping in clinical education: A quantitative score derived from a survey of internal medicine teaching faculty. *Teach Learn Med.* 2019;31(1):53–64. doi:10.1080/10401334.2018.1481752.
22. Tran K, Morra D, Lo V, Quan SD, Abrams H, Wu RC. Medical students and personal smartphones in the clinical environment: the impact on confidentiality of personal health information and professionalism. *J Med Internet Res.* 2014;16(5):e132. doi:10.2196/jmir.3138.
23. Maslach Burnout Inventory (MBI)—Assessments, Tests; Mind Garden. https://www.mindgarden. com/117-maslach-burnout-inventory. Accessed February 11, 2020.

24. Duncan TGG, Mckeachie WJ. The making of the motivated strategies for learning questionnaire. *Educ Psychol*. 2005;40(2):117–128. doi:10.1207/s15326985ep4002_6.

25. Artino AR, La Rochelle JS, Durning SJ. Second-year medical students' motivational beliefs, emotions, and achievement. *Med Educ*. 2010;44(12):1203–1212. doi:10.1111/j.1365-2923.2010.03712.x.

26. Bloch R, Norman G. Generalizability theory for the perplexed: a practical introduction and guide: AMEE Guide No. 68. *Med Teach*. 2012;34:960–992. doi:10.3109/0142159x.2012.703791.

27. Violato C, Hecker KG. How to use structural equation modeling in medical education research: a brief guide. *Teach Learn Med*. 2007;19(4):362–371. doi:10.1080/10401330701542685.

28. Mccoach DB, Gable RK, Madura JP. *Instrument Development in the Affective Domain: School and Corporate Applications*. 3rd ed. New York: Springer; 2013.

29. LaDonna KA, Taylor T, Lingard L. Why open-ended survey questions are unlikely to support rigorous qualitative insights. *Acad Med*. 2018;93(3):347–349. doi:10.1097/ACM. 0000000000002088.

30. O'Brien BC, Ruddick VJ, Young JQ. Generating research questions appropriate for qualitative studies in health professions education. *Acad Med*. 2016;91(12):e16. doi:10.1097/ACM. 0000000000001438.

31. American Psychological Association. Publication manual of the american psychological association: the official guide to apa style. Washington, DC: American Psychological Association; 2019.

32. Lingard L. Does your discussion realize its potential? *Perspect Med Educ*. 2017;6(5):344–346. doi:10.1007/s40037-017-0377-6.

33. Centers for Disease Control and Prevention National Health Interview Survey: Paradata file description. ftp://ftp.cdc.gov/pub/Health_Statistics/NCHS/Dataset_Documentation/NHIS/2018/srvydesc_para-data.pdf. 2019. Accessed February 15, 2020.

34. Popkin G. Data sharing and how it can benefit your scientific career. *Nature*. 2019;569(7756):445–447. doi:10.1038/d41586-019-01506-x.

35. Council NR. *Nonresponse in Social Science Surveys*. Washington, DC: National Academies Press; 2013. doi:10.17226/18293.

36. Artino Jr AR, La Rochelle JS, Dezee KJ, Gehlbach H. Developing questionnaires for educational research: AMEE Guide No. 87. *Med Teach*. 2014;36:463–474. doi:10.3109/0142159x.2014.889814.

37. Gehlbach H, Brinkworth ME. Measure twice, cut down error: a process for enhancing the validity of survey scales. *Rev Gen Psychol*. 2011;15(4):380–387. doi:10.1037/a0025704.

38. Gehlbach H, Artino AR. The Survey Checklist (Manifesto). *Acad Med*. 2018;93(3):360–366. doi:10.1097/ACM. 0000000000002083.

39. Yudkowsky R, Park YS, Downing SM. *Assessment in Health Professions Education*. 2nd ed. New York: Routledge; 2020.

40. American Educational Research Association; American Psychological Association; National Council on Measurement in Education; Joint Committee on Standards for Educational and Psychological Testing. *Standards for Educational and Psychological Testing*. Washington, DC: American Educational Research Association; 2014.

41. Kane MT. An argument-based approach to validity. *Psychol Bull*. 1992;112:527–535.

Concluding Thoughts

Andrew W. Phillips, MD, MEd ■ Steven J. Durning, MD, PhD ■
Anthony R. Artino, Jr., PhD

Surveys are ubiquitous in health professions education. Educators, researchers, and administrators frequently write and complete surveys. There is a long-standing and ever-emerging science to survey design that this book introduces the reader to, using a six-step method with practical examples and lessons learned throughout. Our surveys should incorporate this science because a proper survey is a scientific instrument.

The aforementioned six steps are essential to produce a tool that has the potential to accurately reflect respondents' thoughts, opinions, attitudes, and experiences in a way that can meaningfully influence understanding and change in health professions education and research.

Without a **Needs Assessment (Step 1)**, survey designers run the risk of missing their target question(s) and creating items that are not relevant to stakeholders and do not contribute to knowledge about the phenomena under study. Because the risk of poor **Survey Construction (Step 2)** is high, especially when designers create items with obscured meaning and statistically significant aberrations, it is critical to test the items and **Establish Evidence (Step 3)**. All of that is necessary before **Survey Delivery (Step 4)** and **Data Analysis (Step 5)** can ever take place. Finally, the **Reporting Guidelines (Step 6)** ensure all the prior steps are interlocked and clearly articulated, which results in not only a complete description of the results but also an account of the development process, validation efforts, and how the survey was administered.

Important themes in this book have been the extent to which the steps are interconnected and the flexibility required of designers to adjust as needed for the specific context of a given survey. The purpose of the six steps and inclusion of the checklists at the end of each chapter are not to prescribe *what to do* as much as to prescribe *what to consider*. The choices made for each of the steps and checklist points will vary with every survey project, but the process of considering prior instruments, considering validity evidence, etc. is the constant.

Another important theme is transparency. Because there are so many decisions for which a "right" or "wrong" answer does not exist, the best answer is always to be transparent about not only the decision made but why. Conveying details from survey conception to reporting decisions (including, for example, prior instruments evaluated, validity evidence for the current survey, response rate and nonresponse bias calculations, and statistical approaches) in such a way that the data collection can be replicated allows other survey designers to build on prior work and provides a deeper understanding of a particular construct than a partially reported effort might provide.

A crucial final thought is the notion that there is no such thing as a "simple survey" that will have much value to educators and researchers. If the data are to be used to inform understanding or decisions in any way, the data should be gathered by the best tool available or developed. Every survey worth doing is a survey worth doing correctly through the application of a systematic process, like the steps presented here. We believe that bad data can be worse than no data.

We hope this book proves helpful as a starting point for novice survey designers to take the theoretical and produce a useful instrument and that it serves as a quick reference for experienced survey designers to double-check the complete process of survey design.

Example Worksheet for Study Planning

Title: [study title encompassing its theme]

Question: [research question, often relates to a whole scale]

1. **Measurements**
   a. Subjective method(s): [surveys, interviews, focus groups, and other qualitative, subjective study methods; may be more than one]
   b. Objective method(s): [quasi-experiments, observational studies of numerical outcomes (e.g., course grades), and other quantitative methods; may be more than one]
   c. Possible confounders: [demographics, personal histories, location, and other contextual variables that must be accounted for in any subjective and objective measurements]
   d. Outcome measurement(s): [scales, specific items of interest, course grades, and any other variables that will be measured as dependent variables]
   e. Statistical test: [predetermined approach and tests for variables of interest]

2. **Group Selection**
   a. Sample size necessary: [power analysis based on statistical tests chosen]
   b. Sampling frame: [demographics, historical variables, and any other variables that define inclusion criteria]
   c. Exclusions: [demographics, historical variables, and any other variables that define exclusion criteria]
   d. Control characteristics: [if applicable, defines the baseline against which the intervention group is tested]

3. **Logistical Designs** (for studies with interventions such as a new curriculum)
   a. All Groups: [study protocols that all participants receive]
   b. Treatment Group: [study protocols that only participants in the treatment group receive]
   c. Control Group: [study protocols that only participants in the control group receive]

4. **Database Searches:** [list of searched databases for background information; a separate document should keep track of searches and findings]

5. **Prior Instrument Searches**: [list of searched databases and hand-tracing search for prior instruments; a separate document should keep track of searches, findings, and pros and cons of the prior instruments for use]

6. **Keywords:** [list of keywords both initially attempted and additional keywords discovered during the iterative search process]

7. **Additional Notes:**

Survey Design Checklist[1]

For <u>formulating survey items</u>:

Does your survey...	Yes	No
...avoid formatting items as statements with agree/disagree response options, and *instead*...?		
...use questions with construct-specific response options (e.g., if asking about *confidence*, use confidence in the question: "How confident are you that you can take a history on an uncomplicated pediatric patient?")?		
...ask one thing at a time (thereby avoiding multibarreled items)?		
...use positive language (i.e., avoid *un-*, *in-*, *anti-*, etc.) to ease cognitive processing?		
...avoid "reverse-scored" items (i.e., items in a survey scale whose valence is the opposite of the other items in the scale)?		
...use item formats that answer the question of interest (i.e., a ranking question might be more appropriate than a rating question if the goal of the question is to identify the most and least preferred items on a list)?		
...use the active voice (i.e., the active voice tends to be clearer than the passive voice)?		
...avoid inappropriate assumptions (i.e., assumptions about respondents' knowledge or their living and working situations that may not be true)?		

For <u>crafting response options</u>:

Does your survey...	Yes	No
...use an appropriate number of response options (5–7 options are usually sufficient for Likert-type items)?		
...match the question stem with the response options (i.e., ensure there is parallelism between the wording of the question stem and the wording of the response options)?		

Does your survey...	Yes	No
...include labels for all response options?		
...use only verbal labels (numbered response options are typically not needed, nor are they useful for respondent comprehension)?		
...maintain even spacing in the response options and balance the visual, numeric, and conceptual midpoints?		
...avoid the use of vague response options (i.e., response options that are subject to multiple interpretations)?		
...avoid the use of overlapping response options?		
...provide response options in only one row or only one column?		

For **formatting and organizing the whole survey**:

Does your survey...	Yes	No
...make the first item a relatively easy-to-answer, interesting question that applies to all respondents?		
...ask the more important items earlier in the survey?		
...include instructions that are clear, concise, consistent, and not overly complicated?		
...include only items that apply to every respondent (or employ branching items)?		
...use scales—not single items—when possible (especially for complex topics)?		
...use a consistent visual layout?		

(Adapted from Gehlbach H., Artino Jr. A. R. The Survey Checklist (Manifesto). *Academic Medicine.* 2018;93:360–366 and Willis, G. B., & Lessler, J. T. (1999). Question appraisal system BRFSS-QAS: A guide for systematically evaluating survey question wording. Report prepared for CDC/NCCDPHP/Division of Adult and Community Health Behavioral Surveillance Branch. Rockville, MD: Research Triangle Institute.)

Reference

1. Willis GB, Lessler JT. *Question appraisal system BRFSS-QAS: A guide for systematically evaluating survey question wording. 1999. Report prepared for CDC/NCCDPHP/Division of Adult and Community Health Behavioral Surveillance Branch.* Rockville, MD: Research Triangle Institute; 1999.

Sample Likert-type Response Options

Construct being assessed	5-point, unipolar response scales	7-point, bipolar response scales
Confidence	• Not at all confident • Slightly confident • Moderately confident • Quite confident • Extremely confident	• Completely unconfident • Moderately unconfident • Slightly unconfident • Neither confident nor unconfident (or neutral) • Slightly confident • Moderately confident • Completely confident
Interest	• Not at all interested • Slightly interested • Moderately interested • Quite interested • Extremely interested	• Very uninterested • Moderately uninterested • Slightly uninterested • Neither interested nor uninterested (or neutral) • Slightly interested • Moderately interested • Very interested
Effort	• Almost no effort • A little bit of effort • Some effort • Quite a bit of effort • A great deal of effort	
Importance	• Not important • Slightly important • Moderately important • Quite important • Essential	• Very unimportant • Moderately unimportant • Slightly unimportant • Neither important nor unimportant (or neutral) • Slightly important • Moderately important • Very important
Satisfaction	• Not at all satisfied • Slightly satisfied • Moderately satisfied • Quite satisfied • Extremely satisfied	• Completely dissatisfied • Moderately dissatisfied • Slightly dissatisfied • Neither satisfied nor dissatisfied (or neutral) • Slightly satisfied • Moderately satisfied • Completely satisfied

(*Continued*)

Construct being assessed	5-point, unipolar response scales	7-point, bipolar response scales
Frequency	• Almost never • Once in a while • Sometimes • Often • Almost always	
Quality	• Poor • Fair • About average • Good • Outstanding	
Truth	• Not at all true of me • Slightly true of me • Moderately true of me • Mostly true of me • Completely true of me	• Completely untrue • Moderately untrue • Slightly untrue • Yes and no • Slightly true • Moderately true • Completely true

Sample Expert Review Form

Thank you for providing an expert review of the attached survey. The primary construct measured by the survey is intended to be [*insert construct*], defined as [*insert definition*]. Briefly, the study will entail [*insert methods details such as primary and secondary research questions, sampling frame, etc.*].

Please rate the clarity and relevance of each item within the construct of [*insert construct*]. Also, if you have additional suggestions for how to improve the items, please provide those in the space below each item.

(*Note: Another option is to first ask experts to consider the clarity for all your items for a given construct, and then to ask them about relevance. For an example of this, please see Gehlbach and Brinkworth.*[1])

Item 1
[*insert item stem and response options*]

not at all clear	slightly clear	moderately clear	quite clear	extremely clear

not at all relevant	slightly relevant	moderately relevant	quite relevant	extremely relevant

Suggestions for improvement: _____

_____

_____

Item 2
[*insert item stem and response options*]

not at all clear	slightly clear	moderately clear	quite clear	extremely clear

not at all relevant	slightly relevant	moderately relevant	quite relevant	extremely relevant

Suggestions for improvement: _____

_____

_____

Etc...

Missing Items: Next, please think about the survey as a whole and indicate any important characteristics of [*insert construct*] that are not represented or are inadequately represented by the survey items presented above. Please include your rationale as well.

1. _____

_____

_____

_____

2. _____

_____

_____

_____

3. _____

_____

_____

_____

4. _____

_____

_____

_____

5. _____

_____

_____

_____

6. _____

_____

_____

_____

7. _____

_____

_____

_____

(Adapted from Gehlbach H, Brinkworth ME. Measure twice, cut down error: a process for enhancing the validity of survey scales. *Rev Gen Psychol* 2011; 15(4):380–387.)

Reference

1   Gehlbach H, Brinkworth ME. Measure twice, cut down error: a process for enhancing the validity of survey scales. *Rev Gen Psychol*. 2011;15(4):380–387.

Sample Spreadsheet Layout for Qualitative Analysis

Example of simple and inexpensive approach to limited qualitative data obtained in a survey. The appendix pertains to the running example in the Book Introduction. Coding notes for the group can be easily posted at the top. Each row corresponds to a respondent, and the rows in this chart should correspond to the respondent rows recording other data such as demographics and scale responses to evaluate for associations. This is why it is so important to maintain respondent IDs in the sheet. This example also shows how two coders (AWP and ARA, posted at the top of each of their respective columns in this example) can analyze the same responses to evaluate inter-rater reliability. The columns for one coder should be hidden when the other coder is analyzing the data. This format makes it easy to perform a Kappa analysis. Note as well that not every cell matches between coders in this example since there will almost always be discrepancies between coders.

Notes

For all cells, 1=yes, 0=no

Differentiate counseling practitioner types (e.g., MD, PhD, etc).

"Private" counseling = outside HPEU system

ITEM 33

ID	How can HPEU improve confidence in substance abuse confidentiality?	AWP Private counseling	ARA Private counseling	AWP Staff accountability	ARA Staff accountability	AWP Break glass charts	ARA Break glass charts
45as499	private counseling, staff consequences		1	1	0	0	0
rtuy567	we should know that staff will be held accountable		0	0	1	0	0
58daed5	nothing		0	0	0	0	0
jk678g7	my chart should be locked so staff other than my counselor cannot see it		0	0	0	1	1
8hyj6ik	I want my own counselor, not HPEU's		1	1	0	0	0

Quantitative Analyses

Statistical Test	Classification	Indication(s)	Data Type	Assumptions	Notes
t-test	Parametric	Comparing means between two unrelated groups.	Ratio, interval or ordinal.*	Normally distributed SEM. Independent groups.	Cannot use with more than two variables. Cannot use with confounders. Recommended for numbers not in a scale, such as age, weight, number of experiences.
Mann-Whitney U Test	Nonparametric	Comparing medians between two unrelated groups.	Ordinal Ratio or interval that do not meet assumptions.	Independent groups.	Recommended for comparison of Likert-type items.
Paired *t*-test	Parametric	Comparing means between two related groups (e.g., repeated measures).	Ratio, interval, or ordinal.*	Normally distributed SEM. Same group is measured twice.	Cannot use with more than two variables. Cannot use with confounders. Recommended for numbers not in a psychometric scale, such as age or weight.
Wilcoxon Signed Rank Test	Nonparametric	Comparing medians between two related groups.	Ordinal Ratio or interval that do not meet assumptions.	Same group is measured twice.	Recommended for comparison of Likert-type items.

(*Continued*)

Statistical Test	Classification	Indication(s)	Data Type	Assumptions	Notes
Pearson Correlation (r_p)	Parametric	Determine whether two variables are related.	Interval**	Normally distributed SEM.	Recommended for relationships between interval data that are not Likert-type items R^2 represents the variance explained by the relationship between the two variables
Spearman's rho (r_s)	Nonparametric	Determine whether two variables are related.	Ordinal and ratio. Interval that do not meet assumptions.	None	Recommended for correlations between Likert-type items and for correlations between Likert-type items and ratio or interval data (e.g., a Likert-type item and age).
Chi-square	Nonparametric	Compare distributions between two variables or the observed versus expected distribution for a single variable.	Nominal or ordinal.	None (does not need to be 2x2 table).	Recommended for comparison of Likert-type items, especially if stratifying by another variable (e.g., male responses to an item and female responses to an item).

Note: ANOVA, analysis of variance; SEM, standard error of the mean.

*Use of parametric tests on ordinal data is contested but used frequently. Consultation with a statistician is recommended.

**Point-biserial correlation is an exception to this generalization.

cognitive interview: method to test the degree to which respondents go through the response process model with the intent of identifying potential sources of error within specific processes

cognitive response process model: cognitive model that describes the underlying cognitive functions associated with answering items on a survey as (1) item comprehension, (2) data retrieval, (3) data integration into a judgment (and/or estimation), and (4) response reporting

construct: an abstract idea, theme, or subject matter typically operationalized using a survey scale

contingency checking: type of data error checking that seeks to identify data inconsistencies beyond simply valid ranges; it checks for systemic irregularities that might signal invalid data

dichotomous response options: response options for which there are only two possible answers in any circumstance (e.g., alive or deceased)

evidence, consequences: source of evidence in the five sources model of validity that looks at the impact (beneficial or harmful) of the survey on the target audience

evidence, content: source of evidence in the five sources model of validity that evaluates the relationship between the content of a test and the construct it is intended to measure

evidence, internal structure: source of evidence in the five sources model of validity that evaluates the relationship among items within the survey, and how these relate to what is being measured

evidence, relationships with other variables: source of evidence in the five sources model of validity that evaluates the degree to which the relationships assessed are consistent with the construct underlying the proposed test score interpretations

evidence, response process: source of evidence in the five sources model of validity that evaluates the fit between the construct and the detailed nature of performance in which the respondent is actually engaged; simply put, evaluation of how respondents actually comprehend and answer questions

facet (of reliability or generalization): set of conditions associated with an instrument or its administration in which score variation can arise during replication, such as respondents, questionnaire items, stations, raters, instrument forms, or dates of administration

factor analysis: statistical test used to investigate (especially to confirm) relationships between the items in an instrument and the intended constructs

inference, extrapolation: an inference in the four inferences validity framework that the total score or synthesis of narrative data obtained in the testing setting reflects meaningful performance in a real-life setting

inference, generalization: an inference in the four inferences validity framework that the total score of synthesis of narratives reflects performance across the test domain

inference, implications/decisions: an inference in the four inferences validity framework that measured performance constitutes a rational basis for meaningful decisions and actions

inference, scoring: an inference in the four inferences validity framework that the score or written narrative from a given observation adequately captures key aspects of performance

interpretation-use argument: an up-front plan for the anticipated line of reasoning and associated evidence needed to support the validity argument; the interpretation-use argument is the proposal, and the validity argument is the synthesis of actual evidence

item: a single observation (i.e., question) on a survey

item nonresponse: nonresponse from a participant such as selecting "no opinion" for a question or skipping the question (item) altogether but providing responses for other questions

level of measurement, interval: values are uniform in terms of order and differences between adjacent values (e.g., temperature)

level of measurement, nominal: values do not have any implicated numerical value; values function as names or labels (e.g., gender)

level of measurement, ordinal: values have an implied order, but the difference between adjacent values is uncertain or not meaningful (e.g., academic rank)

level of measurement, ratio: same properties as interval values (uniform in terms of order and differences between adjacent values) with the addition of a true zero point (e.g., weight)

Likert response options: response options that provide hierarchal choices of agreement with a statement (e.g., To what extent to you agree or disagree with the statement "I worry about matching in my specialty"? strongly agree, somewhat agree, somewhat disagree, strongly disagree)

Likert-type response options: response options that provide hierarchical choices or ratings but that are not agreement response options (e.g., How worried are you about matching in your specialty? not worried, somewhat worried, very worried)

mean: the "average," an equation given by the sum of the values divided by the number of values

median: measure of central tendency, the middle term when all of the values are rank ordered

mode: the value that is most likely to be sampled; the value of most frequency

nominal response options: response options for which there is not a hierarchical order, and any associated coding numbers have no numerical significance (e.g., country of origin)

nonresponse bias: a meaningful difference in at least one variable of interest between those who responded and those who did not respond

observation: an assessment event such as a single survey or test item, performance at a single assessment station or single total examination score

optimization: circumstance in which respondents are being thoughtful and are working through all four cognitive processes (comprehension, retrieval, judgment/estimation, and response)

paradata: information about how survey data were collected. Providing extensive paradata gives readers better context in which to interpret survey results

primacy effects: source of survey variance caused by respondents being more likely to select those initial items in the list rather than later items when items are listed vertically in a questionnaire

principal components analysis: statistical test used to determine whether the instrument can be shortened by removing less relevant items without a substantial sacrifice in measurement quality

purposive sampling: sampling model in which potential respondents are specifically invited to participate because of their particular characteristics, such as age, positions held, or expertise; it provides a representative, but not generalizable, sample

questionnaire: a self-administered survey

range checking: type of data error checking that seeks to identify responses outside of the valid response options or outside the expected ranges, such as for demographics

recency effects: source of survey variance caused by respondents being more likely to select response options said last in verbally presented surveys such as by telephone

reliability: reproducibility of findings

response rate: proportion of potential respondents who actually responded. Detailed equations exist for specific response rate definitions from the American Association for Public Opinion Research (AAPOR)

sampling frame: the scope of potential respondents from which the sample will be drawn; this may be the same as the population in a very small population, such as a single class at a single medical school

satisficing: the degree to which respondents take shortcuts to conserve mental energy while completing a survey

snowball sampling: sampling model in which participants already participating in a study are asked to identify others who might be willing to participate; it is helpful when recruiting is difficult

standard deviation: value that measures the extent of deviation for a group of values as a whole

survey: any instrument comprising prespecified questions or items designed to sample and produce statistical information about some aspect(s) of a population

survey method: the collection of information from a sample of individuals through their responses to questions

think aloud procedure: method of cognitive interview in which respondents explicitly verbalize their thinking as they arrive at a particular answer choice

unit nonresponse: a potential participant not providing any response to a survey

validation: the process of planning, collecting, and interpreting validity evidence

validity: "the degree to which evidence and theory support the interpretations of [scores] entailed by proposed uses"; operationalized as an evidence-based argument that supports (or refutes) the defensibility of survey findings in relation to the intended purpose of the survey

validity argument: an organized, coherent, honest, and complete synthesis of validity evidence as applied to a specific use of survey results

validity, construct: source of validity in the classic validity framework that addresses the assertion that responses vary as expected based on an underlying psychological construct

validity, content: source of validity in the classic validity framework that addresses the assertion that survey items constitute a relevant and representative sample of the domain being measured

validity, criterion: source of validity in the classic validity framework that addresses the assertion that there is correlation between the survey responses and some (usually hypothetical) "truth" (criterion)

validity evidence: empirical data and conceptual arguments presented to support the validity of proposed interpretations and uses

validity, face: a colloquial term that can refer to content validity but often refers to superficial features that are insufficient for a validity argument

validity inference: as applied to the four inferences framework, key stages during the survey process in which error (invalidity) can be introduced, namely scoring, generalization, extrapolation, and implications

verbal probing, concurrent: verbal probing technique (for cognitive interviewing) in which the interviewer asks questions about the respondent's thought process as he or she responds to each item

verbal probing, retrospective: verbal probing technique (for cognitive interviewing) in which the interviewer asks questions about the respondent's thought process at the end of the survey or the end of prespecified sections

Page numbers followed by "*f*" indicate figures, "*t*" indicate tables, and "*b*" indicate boxes